LOOKING GOOD
from the Inside Out

Tammy Bennett

Fleming H. Revell
A Division of Baker Book House Co
Grand Rapids, Michigan 49516

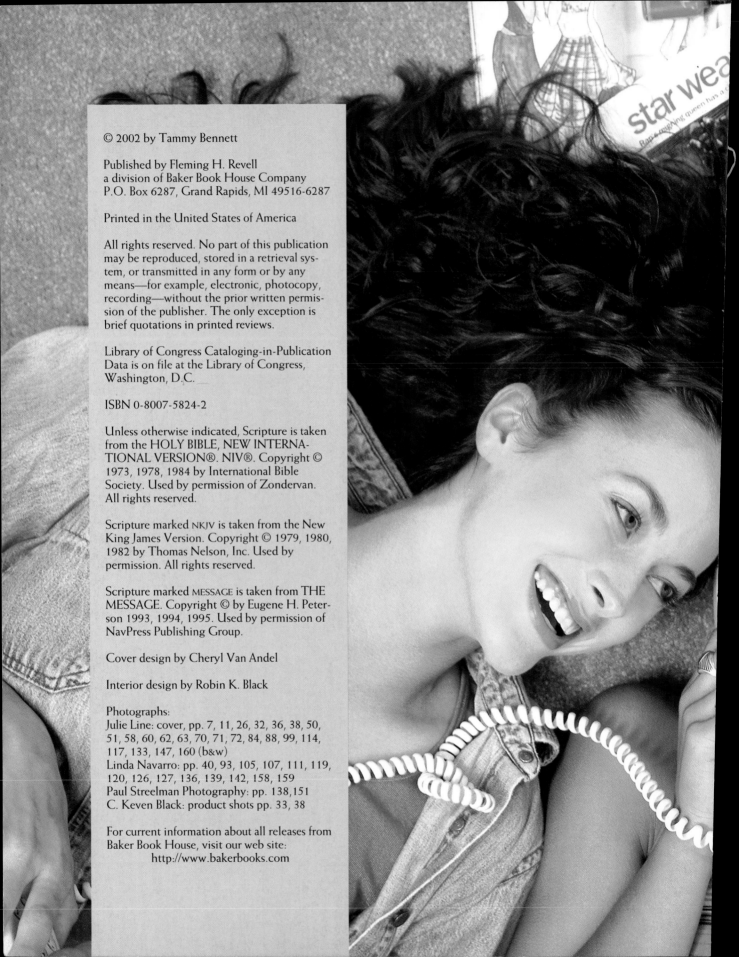

© 2002 by Tammy Bennett

Published by Fleming H. Revell
a division of Baker Book House Company
P.O. Box 6287, Grand Rapids, MI 49516-6287

Printed in the United States of America

Library of Congress Cataloging-in-Publication
Data is on file at the Library of Congress,
Washington, D.C.

ISBN 0-8007-5824-2

Cover design by Cheryl Van Andel

Interior design by Robin K. Black

Photographs:
Julie Line: cover, pp. 7, 11, 26, 32, 36, 38, 50,
51, 58, 60, 62, 63, 70, 71, 72, 84, 88, 99, 114,
117, 133, 147, 160 (b&w)
Linda Navarro: pp. 40, 93, 105, 107, 111, 119,
120, 126, 127, 136, 139, 142, 158, 159
Paul Streelman Photography: pp. 138,151
C. Keven Black: product shots pp. 33, 38

For current information about all releases from
Baker Book House, visit our web site:
    http://www.bakerbooks.com

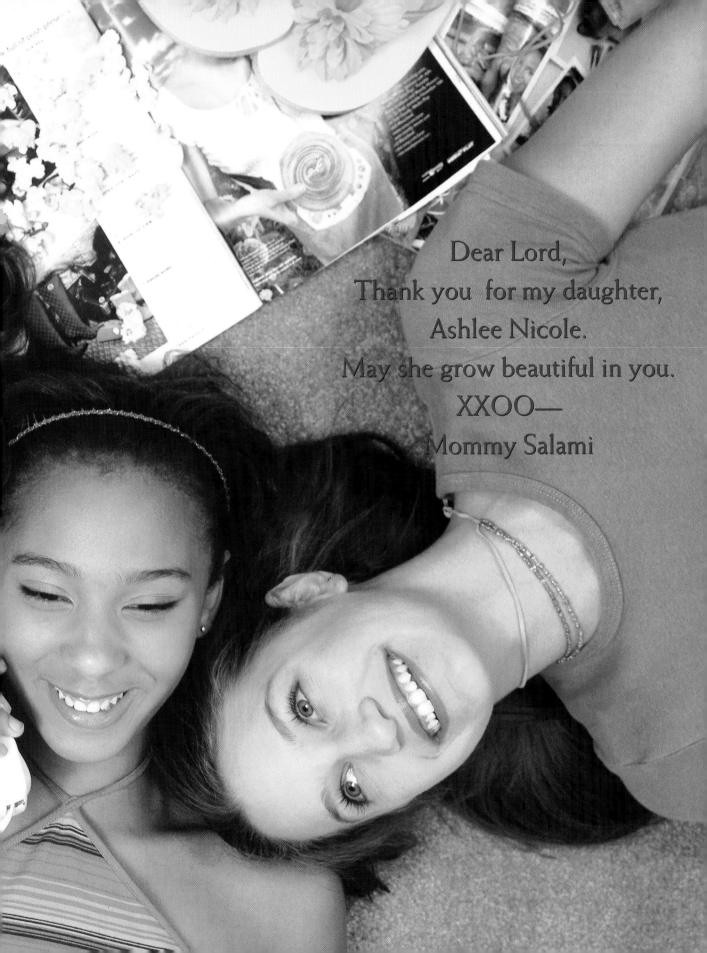

Dear Lord,
Thank you for my daughter,
Ashlee Nicole.
May she grow beautiful in you.
XXOO—
Mommy Salami

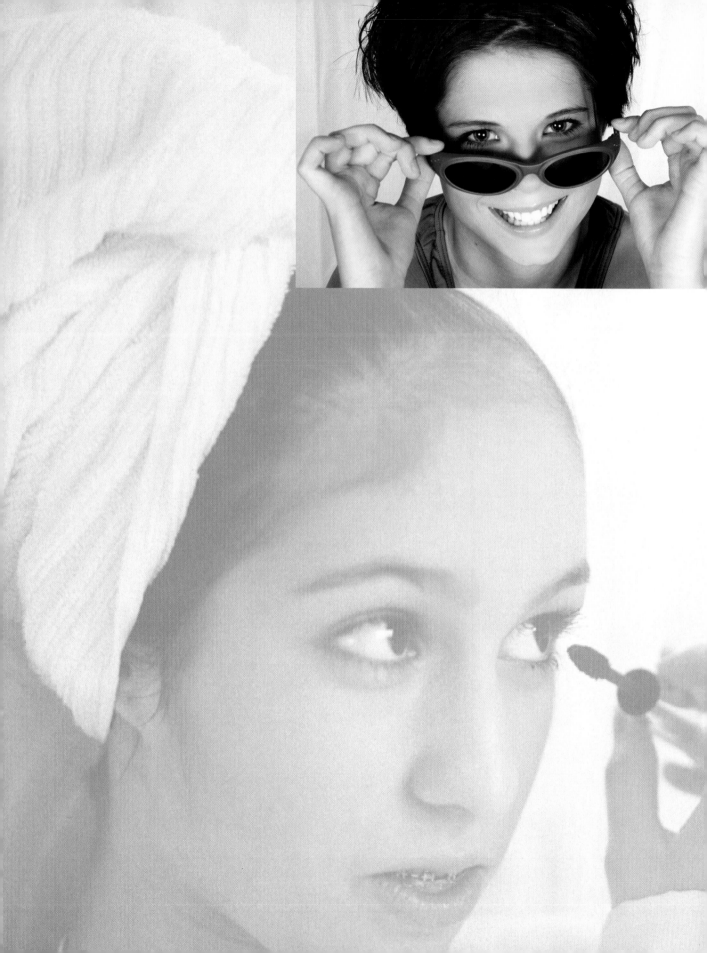

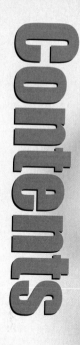

Contents

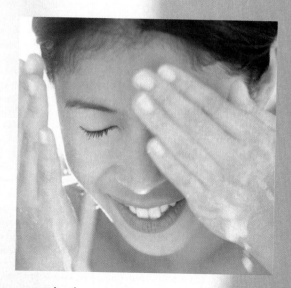

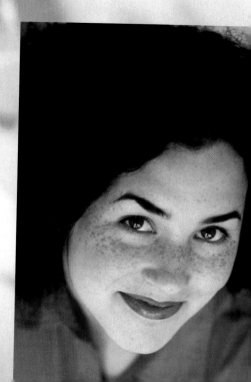

Getting Acquainted

Hi, girls. My name is Tammy and before you get started let's take some time to get acquainted. I won't bore you with too many details. I'll just give you the facts:

- I was a teenager and now I'm not.
- I had a high school sweetheart (Ed) and now he's my husband.
- I had two babies (Matthew and Ashlee) and now they're teenagers.

Now on to why I wrote this book for you.

Like many girls I spent most of my time in hot pursuit of the latest fashions, hairstyles, and makeup. I would flip through magazines hoping to become the girl on the cover, and my wildest and craziest dream was to be Marsha Brady on *The Brady Bunch*. My greatest dilemma at the time was how to get discovered since we lived out in the country in Indiana. When I was thirteen I thought I was finally going to get my lucky break, because my family and I were taking a vacation to California (where I thought all the famous people lived). I was sure this was the answer to my prayers. We toured Universal Studios and even auditioned for the game show *Family Feud*. But even after all that exposure no one discovered me! Once I got back home I knew it was time for drastic measures. So I sat down and wrote a letter to the producer of the TV show *Eight Is Enough* . . .

> There are many faces of beauty and physical beauty is only a small facet of being a "Super Model."

Dear Mr. Producer,

My name is Tammy and I am 13 years old and I was wondering if you ever thought of changing "Eight Is Enough" to "Nine Is Enough"? Because if you have, I'm the girl for you!

Needless to say that tactic didn't work either. The only thing I received was a friendly form letter saying, "thanks but no thanks" and "good luck in your future endeavors."

Years later I did pursue my Hollywood dream only to find out that it wasn't the glamorous life that I had built it up to be in my mind. It was the time I spent there that taught me what it was to be truly beautiful. The fact is that in the acting business I often ran into beautiful people who didn't know how to act beautiful.

Beauty isn't just about hairdos, pedicures, lip gloss, and stylish clothing. Although we equate all of these with becoming beautiful, let's not forget that true beauty begins inside the heart.

Have you ever met someone who was pretty on the outside and pretty ugly on the inside? Or on the other hand, have you met someone who was genuinely kind but kind of homely? Don't you wish you could combine the best of both categories and come up with someone who's kind of pretty and pretty kind? Well you're in luck. This book is going to help you transform your outer and inner beauty so that you can be the best that you can possibly be!

Each chapter of this book is divided into two parts designed to meet the needs of your body and soul. It's my prayer that once you complete this book, your outer beauty will mirror your inner beauty and you will become a "Super Model" for Christ.

Write to me with comments and questions at MakeOverMin@aol.com

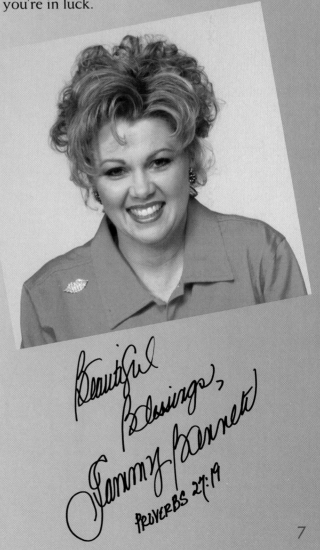

Just as water mirrors
your face, so your face
mirrors your heart.
Proverbs 27:19 MESSAGE

Beautiful
Blessings,
Tammy Bennett
PROVERBS 27:19

7

Skin Care

Cleansing for Your Body and Soul

Everyone wants to be beautiful. When we look and feel good, we can face the world with exuberant confidence, whether at school, at work, or at home. In other words, when you feel better about yourself, others feel better about you too! Since our face is our main point of communication, looking our very best often determines how well we are seen and heard by others. The billions of dollars we spend on makeup proves that we all want our skin to have a healthy glow and our face to look soft, pretty, striking, and stunning. Unfortunately, the cosmetics industry sells gimmicks, hype, and even lies along with the creams and lotions we buy. So before you spend any more money, let's talk about some basics.

The very first step to a radiant, more beautiful you is proper skin care.

When I was a teen I once woke up with a big red zit right at the end of my nose. My face didn't seem to care that prom was just a week away! I scrubbed, steamed, and scalded my face, doused it with alcohol, and masked it with makeup. Nothing worked. That blemish popped right out no matter what I covered it with, and I went through the week feeling like I wanted to hide. I avoided conversations at school and kept my head down with a tissue to my nose, faking a cold. Whenever I heard giggling or whispering, I was sure it was about my hideous red blemish.

The thought of my gorgeous emerald green gown, matching shoes, and perfect pearl accessories didn't seem to make me feel any more beautiful. My prom was ruined.

In high school I thought I was too young to need a skin care program. I figured that was for old ladies. When a blemish did occur on my face, I would feverishly fight the problem with a rigorous skin care routine. When it went away, I quit the skin care until the next emergency. I was in a rush in the mornings and too tired at night to stick with any skin care program. I know now that in less than five minutes in the morning and five minutes at night, I could have avoided some of those problems and much unnecessary embarrassment.

Starting with a fresh, clean surface (your skin) is the key to creating a beautiful work of art (your makeup). Whether you apply makeup or not, starting and ending your day with good skin care is essential to a beautiful face.

A simple skin care program, based on the needs of your skin type (dry, normal, combination, or oily), can refresh your skin and help to give it a healthy glow that will enhance your own natural beauty.

Determining Your Skin's Needs

Let's see what kind of skin you have. Making some simple observations, put a check in the column that best describes your skin:

Check It Out

	Almost Never	Sometimes	Monthly	Weekly	Daily
1. Is your skin prone to pimples?	☐	☐	☐	☐	☐
2. Is your skin prone to blackheads?	☐	☐	☐	☐	☐
3. Do you break out on your back?	☐	☐	☐	☐	☐
4. Do you break out on your upper arms?	☐	☐	☐	☐	☐
5. Do you break out on your chest?	☐	☐	☐	☐	☐

The Answer Is

Check your answers. Use the info below to determine the needs of your skin.

Almost Never–Sometimes—You are blessed to have minor complexion problems. However, even minor blemishes can turn into huge problems when we have to face the world from behind a single zit! You should still follow a regular skin care routine.

Monthly—Your skin tends to be oilier as your body goes through hormonal changes. You will notice a change just before, during, or after your period. Altering your skin care routine during your menstrual cycle can help meet the changing needs of your skin.

Weekly–Daily—Your skin tends to be very oily and needs the utmost care to look its best. While many over-the-counter products work well, you may need to consult a dermatologist. It's money well spent and is sometimes covered by your health insurance. Ask your parents.

Testing Your Skin Type

If you know the special needs of your skin type, you'll be able to avoid products that irritate your skin and waste your time and money as well. Use this simple test to find our your skin type:

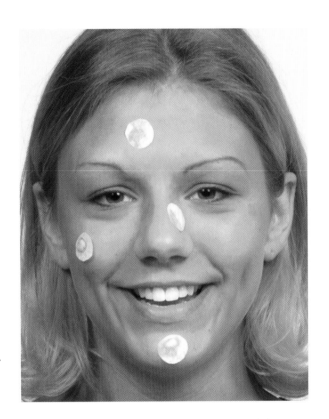

Check It Out

What You'll Need: Perm end papers or curl papers and scissors

Step One: First thing in the morning before you wash your face, take a perm end paper (or curl paper) and cut it into four pieces about the size of a penny. Gently place one of the four pieces on your forehead, one on your cheek, one on your nose, and one on your chin. (The papers will stick on their own from the natural moisture and oils on your skin. If they don't stick, then you know that particular area of your skin is extremely dry).

Step Two: Wait ten minutes and then remove the papers one by one. As you remove them, hold them to the light and examine each one to see how much oil is absorbed from your skin. The dots on the circles below represent the amount of oil found on each paper. Circle the example that best resembles the paper you removed from your face:

Dry	Normal	Oily		Dry	Normal	Oily		Dry	Normal	Oily		Dry	Normal	Oily
	Forehead				Cheek				Nose				Chin	

The Answer Is

What is your skin type? Circle the answer that best describes your skin:

Dry   Normal   Combination   Oily

As a teenager I got very few pimples on my face, but my upper back would often break out with unsightly blemishes of every size and shape. I'd take care of my face, which I could see in the mirror, but I'd forget about my back.

When I showered in the morning I would scrub my back vigorously with a long-handled brush that hung in the family shower. Little did I know that brush was loaded with bacteria that thrives in moist, dark places. Every morning I was making the problem worse by scrubbing bacteria into my blemishes. As my pimples multiplied, it never occurred to me to use the same skin care products I used on my face to help clear up my back. Back then blemish creams came in expensive tiny tubes and just one application on my back would have required the whole tube. Thankfully things have changed today. Now you can buy medicated cleansers made just for your back, arms, and chest area. Along with specially formulated lotions and creams, these products allow you to look your best without spending a fortune!

Dry—If your skin is dry, then you may have had difficulty getting the papers to adhere to your skin. Your paper will have little to no oil on it; however, you may see flakes of dry skin on the paper. Dry skin does not produce enough oil on its own to retain a healthy amount of moisture. Your skin will be tight and flaky. Dry dead skin cells will clog your pores beneath the surface, irritating your skin and causing pimples to form.

Normal—If your skin is normal, it has just enough moisture to make the paper adhere without appearing shiny. Normal skin is a blessing; you should be so thankful to have this skin type. Normal skin produces just the right amount of oils to keep your skin moist without it appearing dry or oily.

Combination—If your skin is combination, it is oily in the T-zone area (forehead, nose, and chin) and normal to dry elsewhere. Combination skin is the most common skin type. Combination skin is oily in the T-zone (forehead, nose, and chin) and tends to break out the most in this area.

Oily—If your face is oily, your paper will be heavily saturated with oil from your skin and your face most likely appears shiny. Oily skin is linked to hormonal changes taking place within your body that produce overactive oil glands. If you have oily skin, your face usually appears shiny no matter how many times a day you wash it. Oily skin is most prone to severe acne problems.

Sensitive Skin

In addition to your skin type, you may or may not have "sensitive skin." Does your skin get irritated easily? Do you tend to break out or develop ruddy, rash-like patches when you apply any type of skin care product to it? If so, you will need to purchase products made for "sensitive skin," available for all four skin types.

Hypoallergenic products usually, but not always, work best on sensitive skin. Always test a small area of your skin first before spending too much money on a product. If you have trouble finding a product that does not irritate your skin, consult a dermatologist.

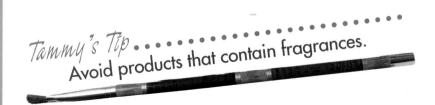

Tammy's Tip •
Avoid products that contain fragrances.

The 4 Steps to Skin Care

The four steps to a good skin care routine are cleansing, exfoliating, toning, and moisturizing.

#1: Cleanser

Cleansing is the first and most important step in skin care. Should you use cleansing bars, foam cleansers, gels, lotions, milks, or just plain old Noxzema to wash your face? Well I'm afraid that's for you to decide based on your skin type. Only you can grade the success of any one product or combination of products over time. You should notice a positive difference in your skin within 5 to 10 days if you are using the right product. If not, try another until you find one that works for you. *Don't give up and don't get discouraged during the search.*

Cleanse your face once in the morning and again before you go to bed. Always use a water-soluble cleanser unless otherwise recommended by a dermatologist. Make sure the product is gentle to your eyes and has no adverse side effects. If it does, immediately discontinue use and try another product, or consult a dermatologist. With your fingertips, gently massage the cleanser into your face and along your jawline. Rinse thoroughly by splashing water over your face several times or until all the cleanser is removed.

Dry—Choose water-soluble cleansing milk formulated for dry skin.
Dry skin cleansers contain light emollients (medicated ingredients that soften and smooth) that leave your skin feeling soft and smooth without feeling greasy.

Normal—Choose a water-soluble cleansing lotion formulated for normal skin. It should leave all areas of your skin feeling clean and refreshed, never tight or greasy.

Combination—Choose a water-soluble, oil-free cleanser formulated for combination skin. When you wash your face concentrate on the T-zone area.

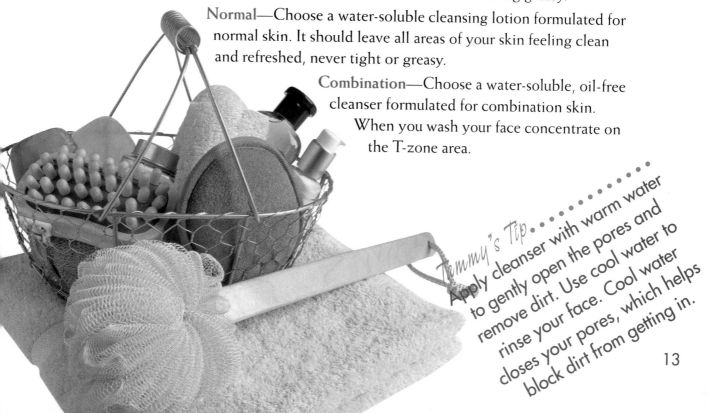

Tammy's Tip • • • • • Apply cleanser with warm water to gently open the pores and remove dirt. Use cool water to rinse your face. Cool water closes your pores, which helps block dirt from getting in.

13

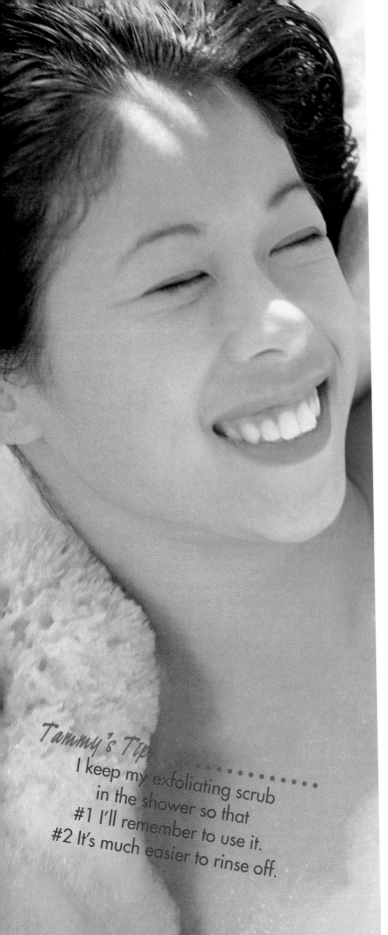

Oily—Choose a water-soluble cleanser that contains 2 percent salicylic acid that will loosen the oil and bacteria from your pores so it rinses easily from your skin. For blemishes or acne, use a cleanser containing 3 to 5 percent benzoyl peroxide. More benzoyl peroxide for more drying and less for less drying. Follow up with blemish cream that contains benzoyl peroxide. Apply it directly on the blemish.

#2: Exfoliator

Exfoliants or facial scrubs are cleansers that contain a fine gritty substance formulated to remove dead skin cells from the skin's surface and expose fresh, new, healthy skin. Old layers of surface skin can clog your pores, trapping dirt and sweat and making your skin much more susceptible to blemishes. *Exfoliating your face twice a week gives you the same results as expensive facials.* Using your fingertips in a circular motion, gently massage the product into your already dampened skin. This will buff your skin without irritating it. Rinse well by splashing water over your face several times until you no longer feel any of the cleanser. Gently blot dry. Apply moisturizer immediately to protect the healthy new skin cells that are now exposed. Never use exfoliants on the delicate skin around your eyes.

Tammy's Tip
I keep my exfoliating scrub in the shower so that
#1 I'll remember to use it.
#2 It's much easier to rinse off.

Dry—Use a buffing cream to loosen dry skin cells and slough off flaky dry skin. Be gentle so you don't pull, stretch, or irritate your skin.

Normal—Exfoliating masks are great for normal skin. Gently massage it in with your fingertips, leave on (follow directions on the product label), and rinse off.

Combination—Use exfoliating masks or scrubs for normal to oily skin types.

Oily—Use an exfoliant that contains AHA (alpha hydroxy acid). AHA helps dry oily skin. Avoid harsh scrubbing that will open blemishes, spread bacteria, and make the problem worse.

#3: Toner

Toner is like the rinse cycle in your washing machine. It continues the cleaning process by lifting and removing any residual dirt or dead skin cells missed by the cleanser. It also restores the skin to its natural pH level (acid level that helps repel bacteria from the skin's surface). Don't use toner around the sensitive eye area, and always apply toner with a cotton ball or pad.

You might want to keep a bottle of toner and cotton balls, or an over-the-counter jar of astringent pads, in your PE locker to freshen up your face after sweating. Good old-fashioned sweat is one of your skin's ways of natural cleansing. Perspiration releases dirt from your pores, and it's a good time to apply a refreshing toner. Your skin will love you for it!

Tammy's Tip • • • • • • • Don't forget to apply moisturizer to your neck. You don't want to have a great-looking face attached to a sagging neck.

Dry to Normal Skin—Avoid toners that contain alcohol that will further dry your skin. Look for toners containing witch hazel. Witch hazel soothes the skin. Use once in the morning before you apply moisturizer.

Combination or Oily Skin—Use a toner that contains alcohol. Alcohol will dry up oily skin. For best results use toner once in the morning and once at night before you apply moisturizer.

#4: Moisturizer

After you cleanse, exfoliate, or tone your skin, it's time to moisturize. Moisturizers don't actually sink beneath your skin's surface, but they do act as an invisible barrier to keep your body's natural moisture from escaping. Moisturizers come in many varieties, from oil-free gels to oily

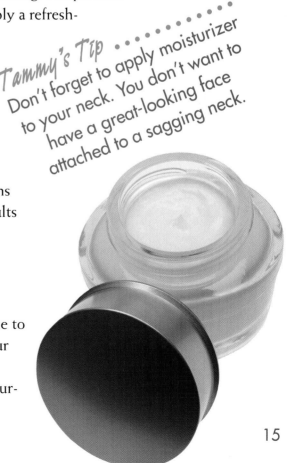

lotions. Based on your skin type and the changing needs throughout the month, you might need more than one moisturizer. In the cold, dry months many of us need heavy lotion to help keep our skin from getting dry and flaky. During the summer months, and often during your menstrual cycle when skin is oilier, you will only need a lightweight, oil-free product. Remember that everyone's skin is different, so what works for your friend may not work for you.

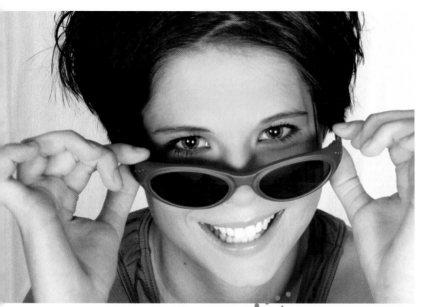

Use specially formulated eye creams or gels for the delicate area around your eyes. These lotions will remove puffiness and smooth out the eye area without irritating your skin. Application of eye creams requires a gentle touch. Using your pinky finger, gently pat the moisturizer on your skin. Make sure you select moisturizers that contain sunscreen!

Tammy's Tip • • • • • When I'm outside and don't want the heaviness of makeup, I tint my moisturizer or sunscreen with foundation before I apply it.

Dry—Dry skin needs a moisturizer that contains heavy emollients. If you have specific areas of your face that are much drier than other areas, then you may want to use two moisturizers: a heavy moisturizer for those targeted areas and a lighter moisturizer over the rest of your face and neck.

Normal—For normal skin apply a lightweight oil-free moisturizer that doesn't feel heavy or make your skin feel greasy.

Combination—Choose two different types of moisturizers to balance the two different needs of your skin. Use a lightweight oil-absorbing formula on your T-zone area and an oil-free moisturizer on the rest of your face and neck.

Oily—Don't skip this step. Many people think that because their face is oily they don't need to use moisturizer because it will just get oilier. However, this is not true. Your skin needs adequate moisture to be its healthiest and to combat acne. Oily skin responds best to lightweight oil-free, oil-absorbing lotions or gels that moisturize your skin without adding additional oils. Another product that works well on oily skin is hydrating mists. In cases of acute acne it is best to consult a dermatologist.

Beauty Bonus

There are several other factors that can adversely affect your skin. Are any of these things you need to address?

Sun—Even a good skin care regimen won't completely counteract the negative effects of too much sun. Sun can cause irregular pigmentation, permanent spotting, and premature wrinkling . . . not to mention various forms of skin cancer. Dermatologists recommend an SPF (sun protection factor) of at least 15 for the optimum benefit. Make sure the product you purchase protects from both UVA and UBA rays. You should use sunblock not only on your face, but also on every other part of your body that is exposed. Not only will this protect from sun damage, it will help to keep your skin moisturized all over.

Diet—A balanced diet is critical to your overall physical development. Both lack of good nutrients and fluctuating weight are detrimental to beautiful skin. Vitamins and minerals are necessary for the natural repair and replacement of healthy skin cells. Every time you gain weight your skin has to stretch to keep up. When you're young, your skin is more elastic; as you age, elasticity is lost and you're likely to be left with sagging skin and stretch marks. A well balanced diet is a key factor in preserving the appearance of your skin.

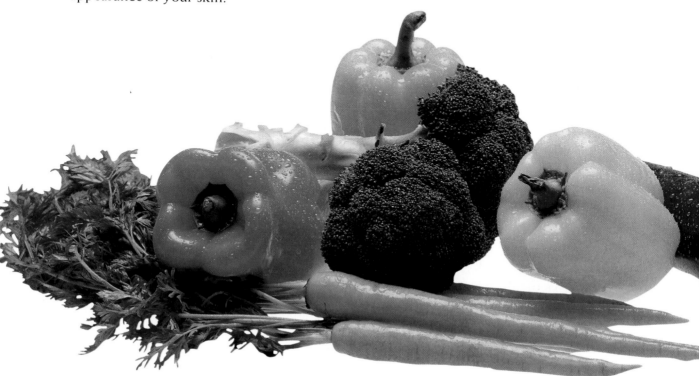

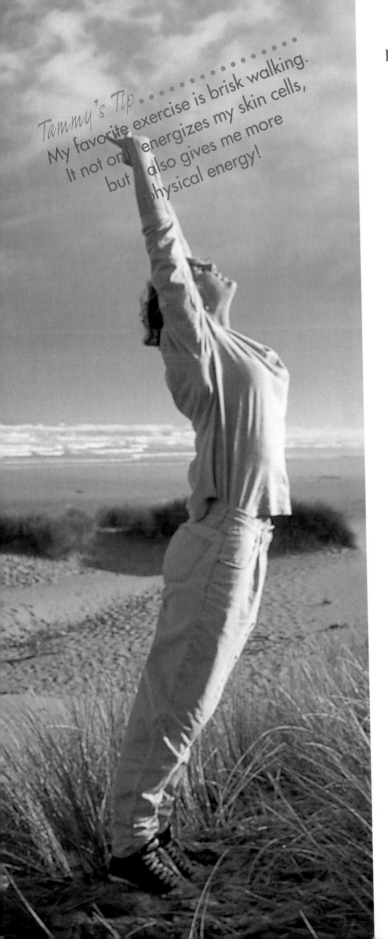

Exercise—Although we often dread it, we need exercise to maintain healthy skin. Just twenty minutes (That's only 50 seconds out of each hour in a twenty-four hour day) of aerobic exercise a day increases blood flow and supplies oxygen to your skin cells, helping to keep that healthy glow. Exercise also helps keep your weight stable, stimulates the sweat glands, which keep your skin clean, and releases chemicals (pheromones) that make you feel revitalized! Exercise can be anything such as jogging, rollerblading, or playing volleyball with your friends.

Sleep—Not getting enough sleep robs your body of the ability to properly nourish and repair all systems, including your skin. When you don't get enough sleep your eyes can be puffy, your skin can be sallow, and your eyes hollow with dark circles. Make sure you get at least 8 to 10 hours of sleep every night. Don't think that you can pull an all-nighter and catch up on your sleep later. It doesn't work that way. You can never catch up on lost sleep. Follow a regular sleep pattern to keep yourself looking and feeling great.

Hormones—Your menstrual cycle is constant fluctuation of hormones, which can affect your mood, your weight, and especially your skin. During that time of month avoid eating greasy foods and wearing heavy makeup. Try a light-weight foundation followed by a light dusting of translucent powder to combat oily shine.

Smoking—Although some people think it looks "cool," smoking stinks. Not only does it rob your skin of much-needed oxygen, it gives you bad breath, the smell stays on your skin, hair, and clothes, and it stains your teeth! As you get older little wrinkles will form around your mouth causing your lipstick to bleed out of your natural lip line. Cigarettes are addictive despite what your friends might think. They can cause many forms of lung, throat, and mouth cancer as well as other deadly diseases. *Don't Smoke!*

Alcohol—Any drink with alcohol depletes your body of water, which is needed for moist, young-looking skin. Drinking causes your skin to look red and blotchy, enlarges your pores allowing dirt and grime to get in, and creates little purple lines on your face (broken blood vessels). Alcohol is fattening. Ever heard the term "beer belly"? Chemically, alcohol is a form of sugar, which is not efficiently used by the body and can cause rapid weight gain. We've already discussed how fluctuating weight can harm our skin's appearance, not to mention the rest of our body! And on top of all that, alcohol can be addictive and cause fatal diseases.

Water—Drinking eight 8-ounce glasses of water a day not only keeps our bodies flushed of impurities that show up in our skin, it keeps the moisture level high and helps maintain proper weight. Ask any supermodel how they maintain weight and good skin, and while their answers will vary to some degree, they will all be water drinkers.

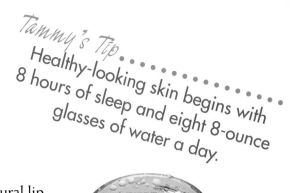

Tammy's Tip ....
Healthy-looking skin begins with 8 hours of sleep and eight 8-ounce glasses of water a day.

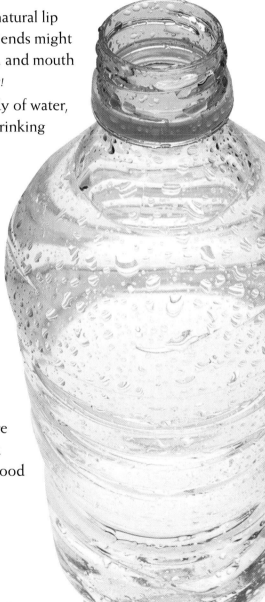

Putting It to the Test

Proper skin care, along with a healthy diet and exercise, can bring beautiful results if you follow a regular routine. Although you might not be thinking about getting older, your aging process started the day you were born! Start taking care of yourself now so that you will look great for all your tomorrows: your twenties, thirties, forties . . . etc.

Track the results of your skin care routine. This will help you determine if the products you are using are effective. If you are experiencing any adverse results, discontinue use immediately and try another product or consult a dermatologist.

My Skin Care Routine

Start Date:_____

Condition of my skin before I get started: _____

Cleanser Name: _____

Results after 5 days: _____

After 10 days: _____

Exfoliant: _____

Results after 5 days: _____

After 10 days: _____

Toner: _____

Results after 5 days: _____

After 10 days: _____

Moisturizer: _____

Results after 5 days: _____

After 10 days: _____

Overall condition of my skin after 10 days: _____

The key to beautiful, healthy skin in the future is a dependable skin care system today.

The key to beautiful skin is good skin care. Even though we wish we had perfect skin without having to cleanse it and care for it, it just doesn't happen that way.

The same that is true for our outer "physical beauty" is true of our inner "soul beauty" as well. We aren't perfect on the inside without soul cleansing. The purpose of this book is for you to become a whole beauty by becoming the best you can be on the outside and on the inside. Whole beauty shines from the core of who we are on the inside, making us appear even more beautiful to others on the outside. It exposes the inner beauty of our soul. Inner beauty begins with cleansing through salvation in Jesus Christ. This isn't a beauty product you find stocked on the store shelves but one that God through his Son Jesus provided for us. There isn't any other beauty advice found in the world that brings true beauty to the surface the way a personal relationship with Jesus will.

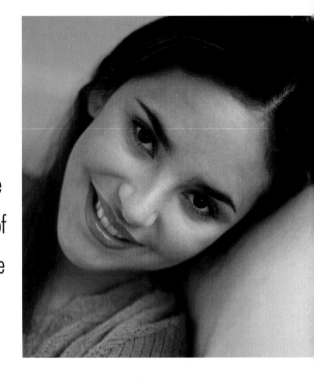

A personal relationship with Jesus imparts beauty to the soul.

Time Out
with Tammy—

When I was in seventh grade I had to move and change schools. We lived in the city and were moving to the country. I hated my parents for moving me away from all of my friends to live in "hickville." I would take long walks in the woods and angrily vent to God about how unhappy I was. Although he was kind of like that invisible friend I couldn't see, I still knew he was there and that he was listening. Did he move me back to the city? No. But he did move a couple of my best city friends to the country. He heard my prayers and answered them in a way I wouldn't have dreamed of. Not only that, I'll let you in on a little secret. If I hadn't moved to the country, I would have never met my future husband. God knew I needed that move.

Inner beauty through salvation in Jesus is an everlasting beauty, meaning that it will never end. Have you ever seen what a former Miss America from 30+ years ago looks like today? You look at her and think, "She's all wrinkled, how'd she ever win?" Well it's like this: Our outer, physical beauty fades with age. We can prolong it with good skin care treatments, makeup, and even cosmetic surgery, but eventually even the most drastic measures won't work. That's what makes inner beauty so unique, it doesn't fade with time; it flourishes forever and ever!

Does this mean you can't be beautiful on the inside without Jesus? Definitely not. There are many kind, friendly, caring people that don't know the Lord Jesus. The difference between their inner beauty and the inner beauty that you receive from Jesus is eternal life.

So why should you be concerned about eternal life as a teenager when your life is just beginning? The soul cleansing relationship you begin now with Jesus will help guide you for the rest of your life. That includes tomorrow and the next day and the day after that. In short, he is the best friend you will ever have. I know it doesn't make sense at first but once you accept Jesus he'll never leave you, and you'll be amazed at how he'll work in your life.

Did you ever have an invisible friend when you were a kid, one that never left your side? Or what about that doll or stuffed animal you shared all your innermost thoughts with? You told them when you were happy, hurt, and disappointed. Could they really be happy, hurt, or disappointed with you? Nope, even though we pretended they were. Well this is the really cool part. Jesus is way better than that imaginary friend, doll, or stuffed animal. *He's for real!!!* He will be happy with you, hurt for you, and yes, even feel your disappointments. And best of all he'll respond to your needs.

Tammy's Tip When it comes to skin care there are many solutions, but when it comes to sin care there's only one solution—Jesus.

So how do you start this awesome relationship? That's where spiritual cleansing comes in. Soul care does for your inside what skin care does for your outside. Jesus washes away impurities and reveals the new likeness you have to him. The Holy Spirit balances your pH (personal hang-ups), and God the Father replenishes your thoughts and desires with those he has for you.

Determining Your Soul Need

So how do you determine the need of your soul? It's not like examining your skin in the mirror each morning and applying the right skin care. It goes much deeper than that. The condition of your soul determines your relationship to God, and your relationship to God determines where you'll spend eternity.

Some people believe that once you're dead that's it, you're gone, you're finished, it's bye-bye, six-foot under pushin' up daisies for you. But according to the Bible, you'll spend eternity somewhere. The question is where?

Romans 6:23—For the wages of sin is death, but the gift of God is eternal life in Christ Jesus our Lord.

The answer to the question comes in the form of a gift from God. Have you ever received a postcard in the mail from a cosmetics counter at your local department

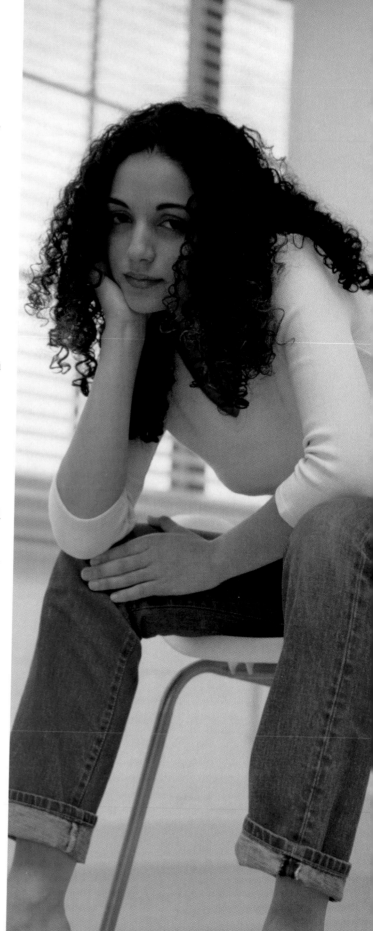

store? It usually reads something like this: "Come to our cosmetic counter for a free gift reserved just for you!"

It's up to you to decide what you're going to do with the invitation. Do you throw it away? Do you doubt it's real? Do you ignore it, misplace it, or even lose it entirely? If you're like most people, you recognize the value of the gift and you make sure you get to the store before the offer ends. The gift is free. Someone else has paid the price for you. When you arrive at the counter to claim your gift, the sales clerk will record your name in their book for future reference. You become a "preferred client."

Did you know that this scenario could be applied to God's invitation for salvation? He sends out the invitation through his Word, the Bible. It's up to us to decide to claim the gift. Are we going to throw it away? Are we going to doubt it? Are we going to ignore it? Each of us has a choice in

Tammy's Tip ••••••••••
God gives you a gift you'll never return. It's just the perfect size, color, and style!

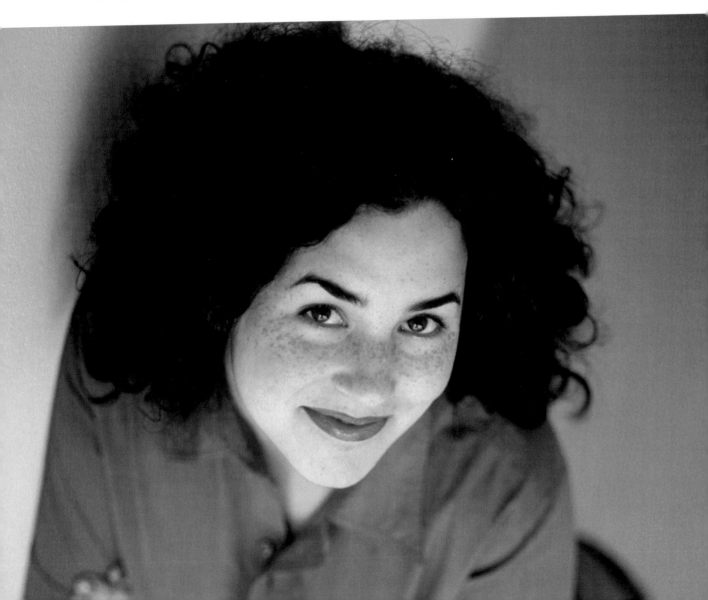

whether or not we will accept the free gift or not. When we claim our present, our name is written in God's "Book of Life." The consequence of *not* taking God up on the offer means an eternity in hell.

Revelation 20:15 (NKJV)—And anyone not found written in the Book of Life was cast into the lake of fire.

Only those who have received the free gift of salvation by accepting Jesus Christ as their personal Lord and Savior posses eternal beauty. Would you like to know how to claim your free gift? The following section is key to the whole beauty process. It's by far the best beauty advice you'll ever apply!

Putting Your Soul to the Test

There's only one way to determine if you're going to spend eternity with God in heaven, and that's by accepting his Son (Jesus) as your personal Lord and Savior. Have you asked him to be part of your life? Not sure? Read on.

The Answer Is

We often find answers to physical beauty in magazines, books, or newspapers; however, to understand inner beauty we need only one beauty manual, the Bible. Check your answers with those found in the Scriptures listed below.

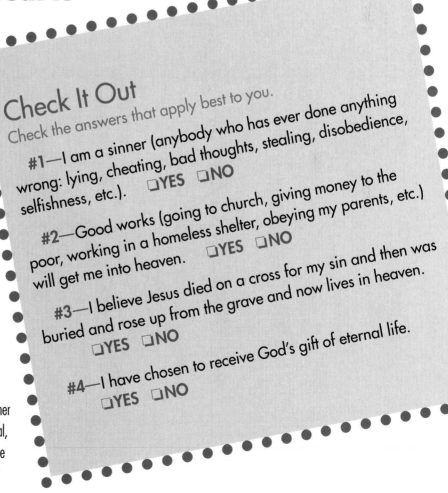

Check It Out
Check the answers that apply best to you.

#1—I am a sinner (anybody who has ever done anything wrong: lying, cheating, bad thoughts, stealing, disobedience, selfishness, etc.). ❑YES ❑NO

#2—Good works (going to church, giving money to the poor, working in a homeless shelter, obeying my parents, etc.) will get me into heaven. ❑YES ❑NO

#3—I believe Jesus died on a cross for my sin and then was buried and rose up from the grave and now lives in heaven. ❑YES ❑NO

#4—I have chosen to receive God's gift of eternal life. ❑YES ❑NO

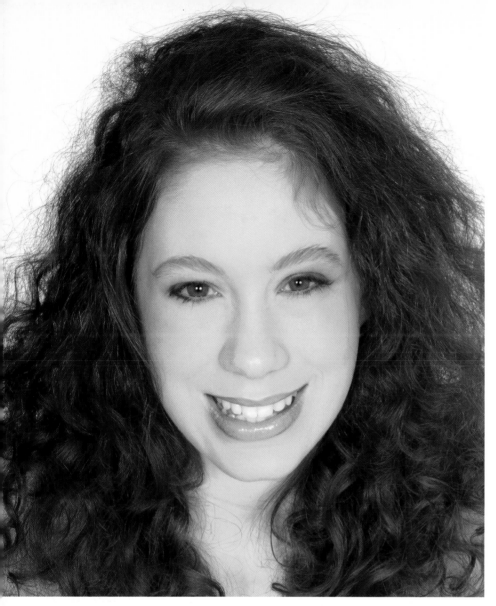

#1—I'm a Sinner

Romans 3:23—For all have sinned and fall short of the glory of God.

A sinner is anybody who has ever done anything wrong. By wrong I don't only mean like robbing a bank or murder. I mean anything wrong: a little white lie, talking back to your mom, gossiping, etc. The Bible says, "All have sinned." You, me, everybody!

#2—Good Works Will Get Me into Heaven

Ephesians 2:8-9 (NKJV)— For by grace you have been saved through faith; and that not of yourselves, it is the gift of God, not of works, lest anyone should boast.

According to Ephesians 2:8–9 there is nothing we do; salvation is a gift of God. Good works will not get you into heaven, so no one has bragging rights. The Bible says, "It is a gift of God." So when someone offers you a present, there's only one thing to do. Accept it.

#3—I Believe Jesus Died on a Cross for My Sin

Acts 16:31—Believe in the Lord Jesus, and you will be saved.

Do you believe it? Do you believe God loved you so much that he sent his Son Jesus to die on the cross for your sins? Do you believe that he was buried and rose again the third day according to the Scriptures and now lives in heaven?

Tammy's Tip
According to the Bible, "All have sinned." And according to the dictionary, "All means all, and that's all it means."

26

To believe we must have faith. Faith believes in something we cannot necessarily see, but have witnessed by all of the physical attributes that are there. I can't physically see the blustery winds; however, I can see the results of them.

Faith means we believe there is a God, even though we can't see him. It gives us hope to trust with our hearts what we cannot see with our eyes.

Now that we've discussed faith, what it is, let's look at how we apply it to our lives. Just like skin care, we have to apply it to experience its effects.

#4—I Have Chosen to Receive God's Gift of Eternal Life

John 3:16 (NKJV)—For God so loved the world that he gave his only begotten Son, that whoever believes in him should not perish but have everlasting life.

God gives each of us free will to choose . . . to believe or not to believe. That is the question. God could have made us all little god-clones with no mind of our own. But he didn't want it that way. God wants true love from us.

What if you could wave a magic wand and instantly become the most popular girl in school by making everyone love and adore you? What fun would that be? Sure it might be fun for a few days, but after that who wants a bunch of phony admiration? God doesn't want it either. He wants the real thing.

> God invites you to accept his free gift of salvation, reserved just for you.

You've just received God's invitation to come to his counter and redeem your free gift. Are you going to throw it away? Are you going to doubt it? Are you going to ignore it? Or are you going to accept it? This is the most important choice you will ever make, and I would encourage you to accept it right away.

The Bible says, "Now is the day of salvation" (2 Cor. 6:2)

When we're young and full of life, the last thing we think about is death. I mean after all, we have hopes, dreams, and plans that need to be carried out. Who has time to die? The possibility doesn't even exist in our minds; however, if we stop and think about it, we really don't have a guaranteed life expectancy.

Time-Out with Tammy—

I used to live in the desert near Palm Springs, California, where it's very windy. Hundreds of windmills surround the area supplying power to the city. Even though I couldn't physically see the wind, I could see the effect the wind had on the windmills as they turned at rapid speeds; and I could see the sand whipping through the air, almost blinding me at times. All of the physical attributes were there even though I couldn't see the wind specifically. The same is true of God. I cannot see God, but I can see the miracles he performs all around me every single day.

Have you taken the time to notice a miracle lately? A newborn baby? An unexplained medical healing? The vastness of the sky, moon, or stars? The intricate growth of a flower or even a blade of grass? The complex detail found in each and every snowflake? All of these, though given scientific definition, are actual God-given miracles.

Tammy's Tip •••••••• Take time to notice a miracle.

I remember when the uncertainty of no tomorrow became a reality to me. It was the summer between my seventh and eighth grade years of junior high school. I was a member of our church's youth choir. We had practiced the "King Is Coming" cantata (that's a bunch of songs put together) for weeks in preparation to sing in churches from Indiana to Alaska. It was to be a major road trip to say the least. At a Sunday evening service prior to the trip we performed the cantata at our own church. I can remember singing through the songs almost flawlessly in preparation for the pastor's brief message at the end. His words struck me funny at the time, but have since haunted me. He said something like this. "We will be leaving for Alaska soon, this may be your only time to hear this cantata. Even though we will present it a second time when we return, this may be your one and only chance to apply it to your own life. For some of you tomorrow may never come." It's chilling as I think back to how those words became reality for one family in the church in particular. Their 18-year-old son would not hear the cantata a second time, because he was tragically killed in a motorcycle accident. His tomorrow never came. His opportunity for decision making was over. Although it was a sad time, we were comforted in the fact that we knew he was in heaven with God because he had received God's gift of eternal life by accepting Jesus as his personal Lord and Savior.

The Most Important Fact

The prayer below is *only* a guide to assist you in communicating your desire to accept God's gift of salvation through his son Jesus Christ. This prayer doesn't mean a thing unless you make it personal between you and God. Anyone can say the words but God knows if the words are sincerely from your heart.

> Dear Lord,
>
> I know that I'm a sinner and that I can do nothing about it on my own, except believe in you. I know that you sent your son Jesus to die for my sins, that he was buried, and that he rose again the third day so that I might have eternal life through him. I accept your gift of salvation by faith and ask you to cleanse me of my sins and be Lord of my life.
>
> In Jesus' name, Amen.

If you prayed the prayer above, I would love to hear from you so I can personally pray for you. Drop me a note at: MakeOverMin@aol.com

The 4 Steps to Soul Care

The four steps to soul care are made easy when we relate them to the four steps of skin care:

#1—Cleansing

Cleansing by accepting God's gift of salvation (that's what we just did in the last section) is the first and most important step of soul care. Without it, the rest of the steps are ineffective. Washing away the dirt on your face prepares the surface of your skin for makeup, and washing away sin provides you with an everlasting relationship with your Maker (God).

1 John 1:9 (NKJV)—If we confess our sins, He is faithful and just to forgive us our sins and to cleanse us from all unrighteousness.

#2—Exfoliating

When we exfoliate our skin, we're removing dead skin cells from its surface, revealing the fresh new skin that lies beneath. Did you know that the same process is applied to our spiritual lives? When you accept Jesus into your life, you become a new person. You have been given a fresh clean start. Jesus gives us new life from the inside out.

2 Corinthians 5:17 (NKJV)—Therefore, if anyone is in Christ [accepted Jesus as their Savior], he is a new creation; old things have passed away; behold, all things have become new.

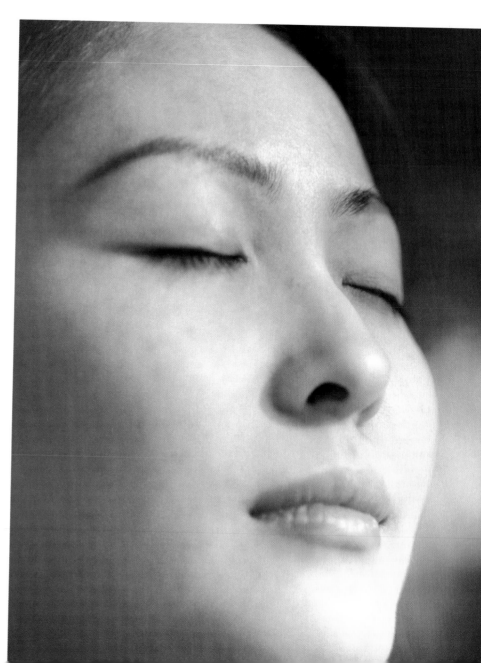

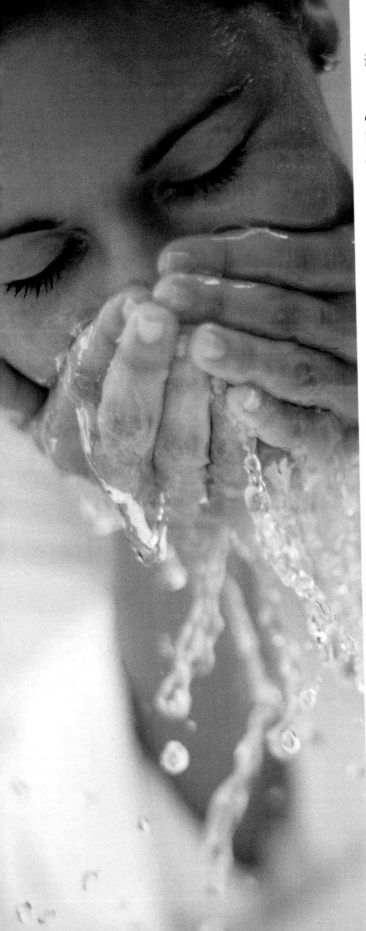

#3—Toning

Toner is used after cleansing to remove excess dirt from our skin and restore its pH level. Once again we can parallel this skin care process to our soul care. When we accept Jesus as our Lord and Savior, the Holy Spirit resides in us 24/7, helping us resist our natural inclination to sin. Like toner, he gets down beneath the surface to the heart of the issue, separating the right from wrong. He levels out our pH (personal hang-ups) by bringing them to our attention so that we can deal with them and move on and become a better person for it. To apply spiritual toner become consciously aware of the Holy Spirit's prompting in your heart and respond receptively to him.

Galatians 5:16—Live by the Spirit, and you will not gratify the desires of the sinful nature.

#4—Moisturizing

Once the Holy Spirit reveals the sin in your life, you may feel like you have an empty void that needs to be filled. For instance, the group of friends you hang out with is into the drug scene. Now that you've accepted Jesus you know that doing drugs is

Tammy's Tip
Don't put off till tomorrow what you should do today!

wrong, but you just don't want to lose your friends. However, you know if you continue hanging out with them, they'll pressure you to keep using. So what do you do?

This is the cool part. When the Holy Spirit convicts us and we surrender to what's right, God comes in like moisturizer and replenishes our lives with what he has for us. He fills the void. The story above is true. And although the girl in this story had a hard time making a decision, she inevitably decided to stop hanging around with them. Shortly after that she started attending a youth group in her area and made new friends. Once she discovered the friends God had for her she was the happiest she had ever been!

Jeremiah 29:11—"For I know the plans I have for you," declares the Lord,"plans to prosper you and not to harm you, plans to give you hope and a future."

Putting It to the Test

Skin care and soul care are the most critical steps in both inner and outer beauty. It's the first and most important step that you can take for yourself in both your spiritual and physical life. To be truly beautiful on the inside, you first must know Jesus personally through salvation, and second, develop your relationship with him. To be beautiful on the outside you first must develop a good skin care system for your skin type, and second, stick with it. Both inner "soul care" and outer "skin care" treatments are necessary to be a "Whole Beauty."

Beauty Secret # 1: Cleansing is the key element to becoming a "Super Model."

Time Out with Tammy—

When I was in high school, my grandpa lived with us. Every morning before my mom got up he'd give me lunch money for school, and then after that I'd go in while my mom was still sleeping and ask her for lunch money. Her response was always the same, "Take it out of my purse." So I did. I didn't think this was wrong at the time. After all if my grandpa hadn't offered, my mom would have had to give it to me anyway. (Isn't it amazing how we can reason anything to our advantage?) One morning the Holy Spirit started convicting me of stealing. Day after day I felt worse and worse about what I was doing until finally I couldn't stand myself anymore. I finally told my grandpa, and guess what? He already knew. He wasn't angry. He just said, "If you need a little extra money, just tell me from now on."

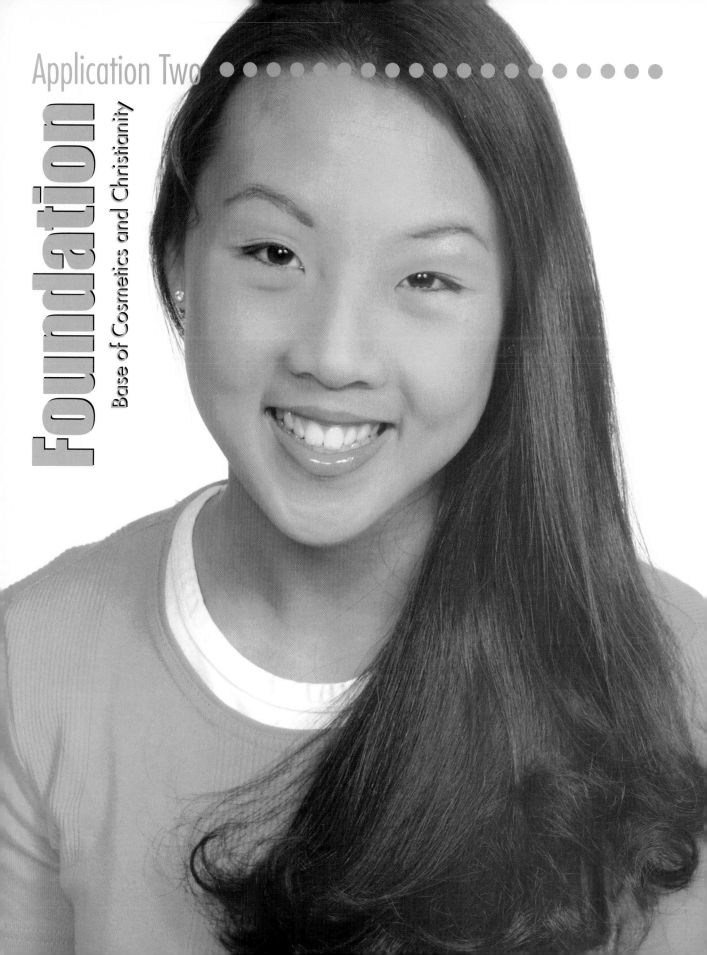

Foundation

Base of Cosmetics and Christianity

After skin care, foundation is the second most important step to creating beautiful skin. Foundation gives a face that porcelain finish that we all desire. The correct foundation will blend the texture and tone of your face, leaving it flawless. The key is finding the right shade and coverage for your particular skin type, texture, and tone. The makeup counters are filled with many different foundations, everything from sticks to water-based formulas. So where should we begin? Let's narrow down our choices by learning what to look for.

Foundation is the most important cosmetic you will ever buy.

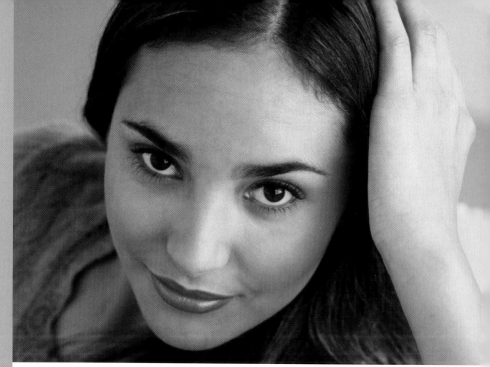

I remember the first time my mom said I could wear makeup. I went to the store in hot pursuit of the basics: foundation, blush, eye shadow, and mascara. When I got there, I stood in a daze wondering what colors to buy. I wanted to look tan, so I bought the darkest foundation I could find. When I got home I eagerly began the transformation process by smearing foundation all over my face. Oops! My neck looked too white, so I spread some there. Then my neckline looked wrong, so I put on just a little more . . . perfect! But after another minute, I noticed how pasty my arms and hands looked, so I applied some there as well. Do I need to tell you how ridiculous I looked when I finished?

Even though I had studied the faces of supermodels in magazines, I didn't have a clue about the needs of my own skin. I could have saved lots of time and money if I would have avoided the expensive trial and error method when learning about cosmetics.

This is the one product we don't want to skimp on when it comes to time and money. The right foundation is crucial to the overall effect of our appearance, including what we wear. Even if the rest of our cosmetics and clothing are perfect, we still won't look our best if we start off with the wrong base.

In this application I'm going to help you avoid the costly mistakes I made. You will learn how to determine the needs of your skin, what types of foundation are available, and how to correctly apply it.

Finding the Perfect Foundation

Choosing the right base formula isn't easy when there are literally hundreds to choose from. This application will give you the three Ts to selecting the perfect foundation: type, texture, and tone. First you need to know your skin type: dry, normal, combination, or oily. Then you need to determine its texture and tone. Remember, if your foundation isn't right, any other makeup you apply will look wrong. But when you apply a good foundation, you're on your way to looking spectacular!

Tammy's Tip • • • • • • • • • • • • • • •
Don't use foundation as self-tanner.

Check It Out

#1: Type

This step is easy because you've already determined your skin type in application one. If you need a quick reminder see page 11.

Circle your skin type.

Dry   Normal   Combination   Oily

#2: Texture

What do I mean by skin texture? Is your skin soft, smooth, rough, pitted, scarred, or acne-prone? The texture of your skin will determine the intensity of coverage you need. Your skin texture may fluctuate with hormonal and weather changes, so you may need to have more than one type of foundation on hand. Examine your skin closely on a regular basis to determine the amount of coverage you need.

Circle your skin texture.

Soft   Smooth   Rough   Pitted   Scarred
Acne-Prone   Other

#3: Tone

Foundation should always match your natural skin color, blending easily into your hairline and jawline. It should improve the tone and texture of your skin without being noticed—after all, you don't want to look like you're wearing a mask. The first step to determining your skin tone is discovering whether it's light, medium, or dark. Light skin ranges from very fair (almost transparent) to a creamy ivory. Medium skin is beige to tan in color, and dark skin includes deep suntan to rich nutmeg shades. The second thing to consider is any skin discoloration that may need extra attention. This will not affect your basic skin tone, but it will affect the amount of coverage you need to look for.

Circle your skin tone.

Light   Medium   Dark

Note any skin discoloration:

The Answer Is

Before you go to the cosmetic counter, do your homework so you'll know what type of foundation to look for. You want it to blend well and compliment the type, tone, and texture of your skin. To help you narrow your choices I've separated several foundation formulas into two categories: dry to normal skin and combination to oily skin.

Dry to Normal Skin

Water-based Liquids: (light coverage) Water-based liquid foundation sounds "oil-free" but it's not. It just contains more water than oil. The oil allows the foundation to blend easily, giving your skin a natural healthy glow.

Tinted Moisturizers: (light coverage) These are great when you don't want to wear makeup but you want added skin protection. They contain a hint of color to even out your skin tone, moisturizing emollients, and SPF 15 or higher for protection from harmful sun rays.

Cream to Powder: (medium coverage) Cream to powder combines the moisturizer of cream with the sheerness of powder to give your skin a one-step matte finish.

Oil-based Liquids and Sticks: (heavy coverage) Oil-based liquids and sticks contain rich emollients that moisturize your skin. Keep in mind that although it will give you complete coverage, it will be more difficult to blend.

Combination to Oily Skin

Oil-free Liquids: (light coverage) Most oil-free foundations contain silicone oils that allow them to spread easily. The oils evaporate, leaving your skin practically oil-free.

Cakes or Powders: (medium coverage) These work well for the gal on the go who doesn't have time to fuss. They absorb oil and prevent breakthrough shine, but beware of caking.

Wet/Dry: (heavy coverage) Sponge on with a damp sponge for maximum coverage or use it throughout the day as a powder to combat oily shine.

Oil-free Stick: (heavy coverage) Foundation sticks provide extra coverage and can double as concealer.

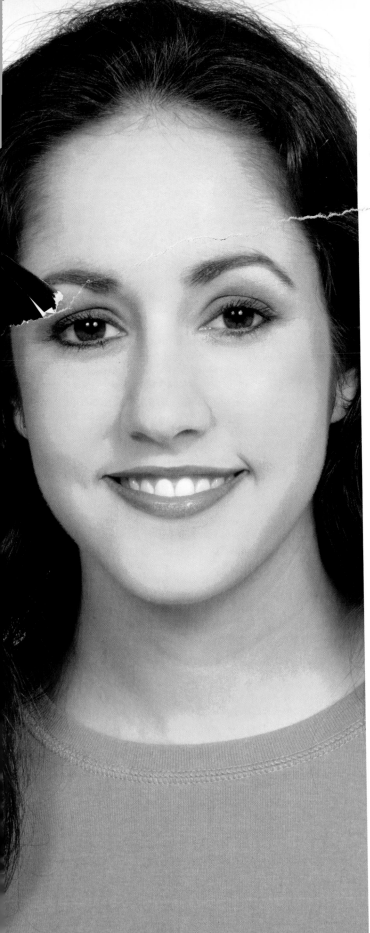

Beauty Bonus

Foundations contain extra ingredients that do more than make us look good. They also benefit our skin. Below you'll find a list of extra helps that certain formulas provide.

Alpha-Hydroxy Acids: AHA chemically moisturizes and exfoliates skin, removing dead skin cells and leaving it smooth and soft.

Hypo-Allergenic: These foundations are allergy tested and work well on sensitive skin. If you have sensitive skin, always read the ingredients before buying a product.

Fragrance Free: These products contain no artificial fragrances that can trigger allergic reactions.

Retin A: This form of vitamin A is used to treat acne.

Salicylic Acid: Foundations containing this beta-hydroxy acid treat acne and keep skin clear.

SPF (Sun Protection Factor): Foundations that contain an SPF of 15 or higher combat the negative effects of the sun's harmful UVA/UVB rays.

Tammy's Tip • • • • • • • • • • •
For ultimate sun protection, apply a facial sunscreen SPF 15 or higher 15 minutes before you apply your foundation.

Putting It to the Test

Finding the right foundation will require time and effort on your part, so be patient. Visit a local cosmetics counter and try the foundation samples before you buy one. You can go to a discount store, but they don't have samples. Ask about the return policy before you purchase anything. You can usually purchase cosmetics, sample them, and return them if they're wrong as long as you have your sales receipt. Remember that cosmetics are an investment. Be a savvy shopper and invest your time and money wisely.

Check It Out

Step One: Before you try anything on, first take it all off—your makeup that is. You want to arrive at the cosmetics counter with a fresh clean face and a small hand-held mirror.

Step Two: Choose a formula for your skin type and texture. For example, do you need a light oil-free liquid or a heavy stick for extra coverage?

Step Three: Select a color that matches your skin tone. Ask for a sample in that particular color, as well as two shades lighter and darker. This will give you five samples to start with. If these don't work, try five more and so on.

Step Four: One at a time, apply each sample to your jawline and blend. Do not test samples on the back of your hand! Seldom are your hand and face the same color.

Step Five: Go outside in the natural sunlight and use your mirror to see if the color you applied is a perfect match. You shouldn't see a makeup line, and it should blend perfectly into your jawline.

Step Six: Once you've found a foundation color to match your skin tone, it's time to check the intensity. Apply to your entire face and see if it gives you ample coverage over your skin texture. If it doesn't, test other formulas of foundation in the same color. If it does give good coverage, bravo! You've found the perfect foundation for your skin!

How It Applies

Now that you've found the appropriate foundation, let's talk about application. The trick to applying foundation is giving maximum coverage without looking like you have any on. It's always best to apply your makeup in natural daylight or a makeup mirror with daylight setting.

Step One: Wash, tone, and moisturize (unless you're using a tinted moisturizer as a foundation) your face. Allow the moisturizer to absorb for ten minutes before you begin.

Step Two: With clean hands, use your fingertips to gently dot your forehead, cheeks, nose, and chin with foundation. Don't apply too much—it's always easier to add more if you need it.

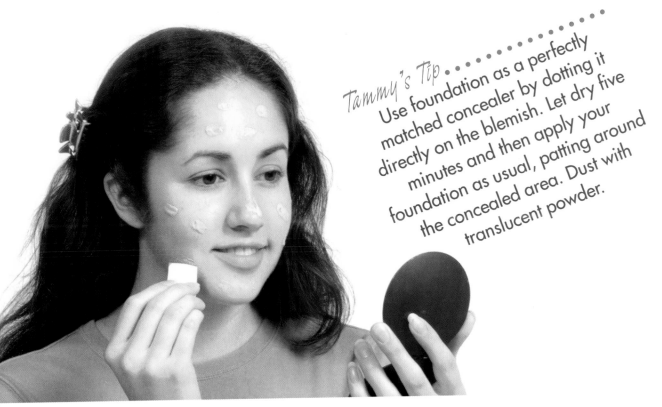

Tammy's Tip • • • • • • • • Use foundation as a perfectly matched concealer by dotting it directly on the blemish. Let dry five minutes and then apply your foundation as usual, patting around the concealed area. Dust with translucent powder.

Step Three: Use a clean makeup sponge to gently smooth the foundation over your face, blending it into your skin so there are no visible streaks or lines. Also blend it onto your eyelids and lips to help your eye shadow and lipstick wear longer.

Step Four: For extra coverage, apply two thin coats of foundation instead of one heavy coat.

Step Five: Check your jawline and hairline to make sure you're well blended. If your foundation is too heavy, blend with a damp makeup sponge or spritz your face with water and gently blot with a tissue.

Step Six: Lightly dust your face with loose translucent powder. (If you're going to apply concealer, add powder afterwards.) This will combat oily shine and keep your face looking fresh all day.

When you artfully apply foundation to your skin, your face becomes the perfect canvas of tone and texture. Now it doesn't matter whether or not you apply other cosmetics because your skin is a beautiful work of art!

Use the following form to measure the success of the foundations you try. Once you have found a perfect match, write the product information in the blanks provided. Cosmetic companies change their product names (especially the color names) quite frequently to keep up with changing trends, but if you know the old product information the company can help you match it to the new products.

The key to great-looking makeup is found in the perfect foundation.

Finding My Foundation

Date:_____

Skin Type:

Skin Texture:

Skin Tone:

How much coverage will you need?   Light   Medium   Heavy

In the spaces below write down the name of the product and the color you are testing. Determine if it matches your skin tone and sufficiently covers the texture of your skin.

1. Product name: Color:
    Does it match your skin tone? YES / NO
    Is it the right amount of coverage? YES / NO

2. Product name: Color:
    Does it match your skin tone? YES / NO
    Is it the right amount of coverage? YES / NO

3. Product name: Color:
    Does it match your skin tone? YES / NO
    Is it the right amount of coverage? YES / NO

4. Product name: Color:
    Does it match your skin tone? YES / NO
    Is it the right amount of coverage? YES / NO

5. Product name: Color:
    Does it match your skin tone? YES / NO
    Is it the right amount of coverage? YES / NO

My Perfect Match

Product Name: Color:

Manufacturer's Name:

The key to great-looking makeup is using the perfect base. When skillfully applied, the right foundation will give us the look of flawlessness even when our skin is less than perfect. Did you know the same principle manages our Christian lives as well? The foundational relationship we have in Christ is an important part of our inner

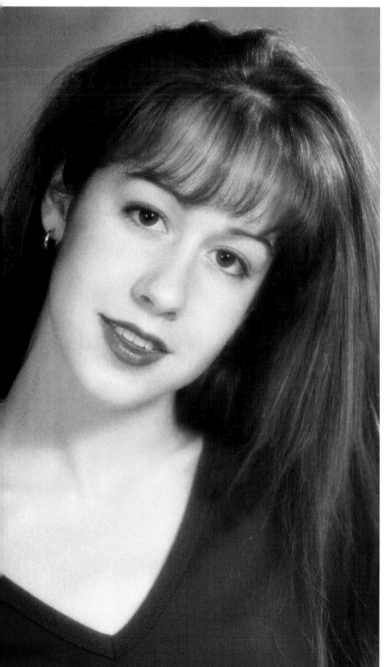

beauty. A solid foundation in Christ will help us deal with life when it's less than perfect. We can apply other things to our lives, but it's like putting makeup on the wrong foundation. Without laying the right foundation first, nothing has the ability to reach its God-given potential.

Building a solid foundation in Jesus Christ is the key to a successful Christian life.

Finding the Perfect Foundation

Everything has a starting point, something to build on. If you're a runner, you exercise, stretch, and build endurance for a marathon. You start out running a half mile, then a mile, five miles, and so on. If you're a basketball player, you practice dribbling, free throws, and layups to improve your game point average. If you're a musician, you learn the basics of theories, scales, and finger positions, and then you practice your music to gain and retain first chair. Anything you do must begin with good fundamentals, a basic foundation that helps you meet challenges.

As Christians, we rely on the same principle. We must learn the basics to shape and mold ourselves in Christ. Then we'll be ready to meet life's challenges head on. In part two of this application, we're going to discuss how to *find*, *apply*, and *build* upon the perfect foundation in God so you can have a *fabulous* relationship with him!

Think about the time you met your best friend. What were some of the things you did to become such *fab* friends? First you tried to *find* out everything about each other. Second you *applied* yourself to the relationship by hanging out and doing stuff together. And you didn't become best buds overnight, because you *built* a better friendship over the course of time.

The same thing applies to our relationship with God. We find, apply, and build!

Check It Out

Find

You've already found Jesus, now find out more about him through prayer, Bible reading, church, and Christian friends.

Apply

Learn how to personally apply prayer, the Word, church, and Christian friendships to your own spiritual growth.

Build

Over the course of time you'll build on your relationship as you trust in Jesus more and more every day!

The Answer Is

Prayer

A remarkable foundation in Christ is found by talking to him through prayer, Bible reading, church attendance, and seeking Christian friends. Prayer is talking to God, just like basic conversation. Often we hear beautiful prayers made up of "churchy" words, which are fine but not necessary for clear communication with God. God just wants us to speak from our hearts. He doesn't expect long lengthy eloquent speeches to flow from our lips; he just wants us to talk to him.

Tammy's Tip The makeup of my foundation is based on a Fab relationship in Christ.

Time Out
with Tammy—

There was a time I hated the thought of praying out loud in front of anyone. I was afraid I'd somehow mess up and be laughed at. I was asked once to pray out loud in front of a group. Before I could answer someone eagerly volunteered and saved me from having to do it. After that, I determined never to be caught off guard again. I went home, composed a prayer, and memorized it for future use. It went something like this:

Dear Blessed Almighty Father God,
Thank you for bestowing bountiful blessings before us. We beseech you to be with us this beautiful day as we boldly bow before your throne of grace.
In Jesus' most precious, holy, glorious name, Amen.

Of course one thing you never want to do is get nervous when you're reciting a prayer. When I tried my prayer out in public, I repeated the first line three times followed by "hmm…hmmm…" hoping the rest of it would come to me. And you know what? No one laughed. I learned from then on just to be myself whenever I talked to God.

God hears us no matter what. It's not the words we use; it's the sincerity behind them. The Bible says that whenever you're praying God's listening.

Jeremiah 29:12—"Then you will call upon me and come and pray to me, and I will listen to you."

Isn't it great to know that we're in touch with a God who cares? He anxiously waits for us to discuss anything with him . . . even guys!

Bible

Bible reading almost seems archaic today. But let me assure you it's never outdated. It applies to us now more than ever. Every answer to every question we have can be found in the Bible. It's the best self-help, how-to guide ever written. Its pages contain all the information we'll ever need to live a full life. The hardest part of applying it to our lives is finding time to read it.

The fact is just like everything else we do, we have to *make* time for it. It's not easy, but once it becomes part of your schedule you'll rely on it. God often gives me a verse in the morning that's just what I need to get through the afternoon.

Psalm 119:105—Your word is a lamp to my feet and a light for my path.

God knows everything I'm facing and gives me the answers I need at just the right time. When I read the verse above, I picture it kind of like a light bulb going off in my head when I read and understand Scripture that applies directly to me.

I've heard some say they don't read the Bible because it's boring. Boring? Never! God is a brilliant author who uses everything from seductive romance (Samson and Delilah) to the detection of premeditated murder (Esther) to teach us lessons about our lives. If sci-fi is your thing, then read about the future in Revelation. Just bear in mind, unlike fiction, the Bible is one hundred percent true!

Tammy's Tip • • • • • • • • • • •
Use a diary to write your prayers to God. This way you can securely pour out the innermost thoughts of your heart to the one who loves you the most.

Church

Allow me to clarify something right from the start. Church is not the building in which you conduct worship. Church is a group of Christians coming together for the purpose of praise, worship, and encouragement in the Lord.

Church shouldn't be the place your parents force you to go, but a place where you look forward to hanging out. It's a great place to socialize with people who know and care about you. It's a place to work with others, study God's Word, and learn more about yourself. Church should be a safe place, a place to fit in and belong.

Matthew 18:20—"For where two or three come together in my name, there am I with them."

God says that if there are as few as two gathered together in his name he is right there in the midst. Wow! What a great place to be—in the presence of God!

Friends

Everyone needs friends. But what type of friends do you have? Do your friends encourage you in a positive or negative way? Do they entice you to do what's right or what's wrong?

1 Corinthians 15:33—Do not be mislead: "Bad company corrupts good character."

Friends play a leading role in our lives. They are often a reflection of who we are. That's why our parents get concerned when we hang out with the "wrong crowd." It's okay to be friendly with everyone, but be selective with who you hang with. If your friends are doing the wrong things and they tempt you to join them, don't hang out with them!

Proverbs 1:10—If sinners entice you, do not give in to them.

Tammy's Tip.........
A great place to start is in a Bible study or youth group.

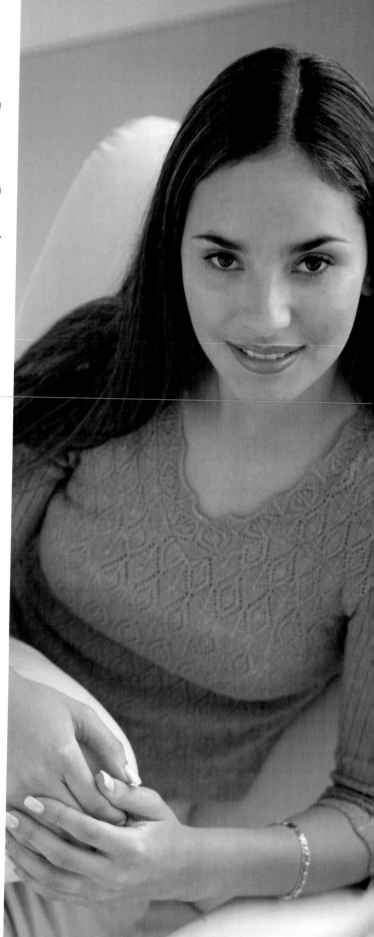

I was friendly with everyone in high school because I craved popularity, but I didn't spend my leisure time with them. I hung out with my friends in youth group, even though the kids in my high school would have considered some of them kind of "nerdy." They were the best friends you could ever ask for. We bowled, roller-skated, swam, sledded, and prayed together. We were free to be ourselves. That's what real friendship is all about—having someone love you for who you are.

You are someone special and you need a kindred spirit in Christ who will truly understand your heart and soul. When I made mistakes in high school, I had friends who prompted me to do better and even prayed that I would. I can't overemphasize the importance of having a Christian friend that will love you no matter what, keep you accountable through thick and thin, and pray for you on a regular basis. If you're in need of that kind of friend, pray and ask God for one.

Proverbs 17:17—A friend loves at all times [through the good times and the bad ones too].

Beauty Bonus

The computer has revolutionized the way we stay in touch through Christian teen web pages. They offer everything from prayer and Bible studies to accountability and biblical advice.

Here is a list of sites to visit:

Brio (my favorite!)—www.briomag.com—Brio is the online equivalent to *Brio* magazine. It covers everything from dating to the latest fashions. Got a question? E-mail and ask their staff of experts for an answer.

Sloppy Noodle—www.sloppynoodle.com—This is an awesome youth site that contains e-cards, movies, articles, music, etc. And it's offered in Spanish and English.

Accountability Online—www.aocentral.com—Their mission statement says it all. "Accountability Online's mission is to provide a safe, fun, and resourceful site for teens to visit, to help teens in their journey with Christ, to save people from the pits of Hell, to keep people accountable to God, and most importantly to lift up the name of Jesus Christ!"

ChristianTeens.net— christianteens.net—With a click of the mouse, ChristianTeens.Net takes you to games, jokes, Q&A, homework help, photo chat, prayer requests, and much, much more.

Tammy's Tip • • • • • • • • Chat rooms are meant to be fun; however, even Christian ones aren't necessarily safe. Never give out personal information such as your last name, address, telephone number, name of your school, credit information, etc.

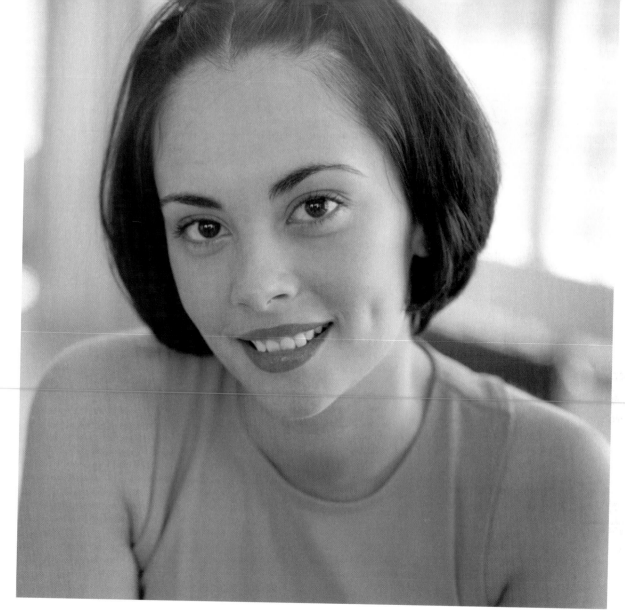

Putting It to the Test

I can give you a lot of information about building your base, but unless you put it to the test you'll never know how well it works.

When you start with the right foundation, everything else will fall into place. Whether it's your cosmetic base or the principles you base your life on, good foundations are necessary to your overall makeup.

Beauty Secret #2: A good foundation is the basis for establishing the "Super Model" in you.

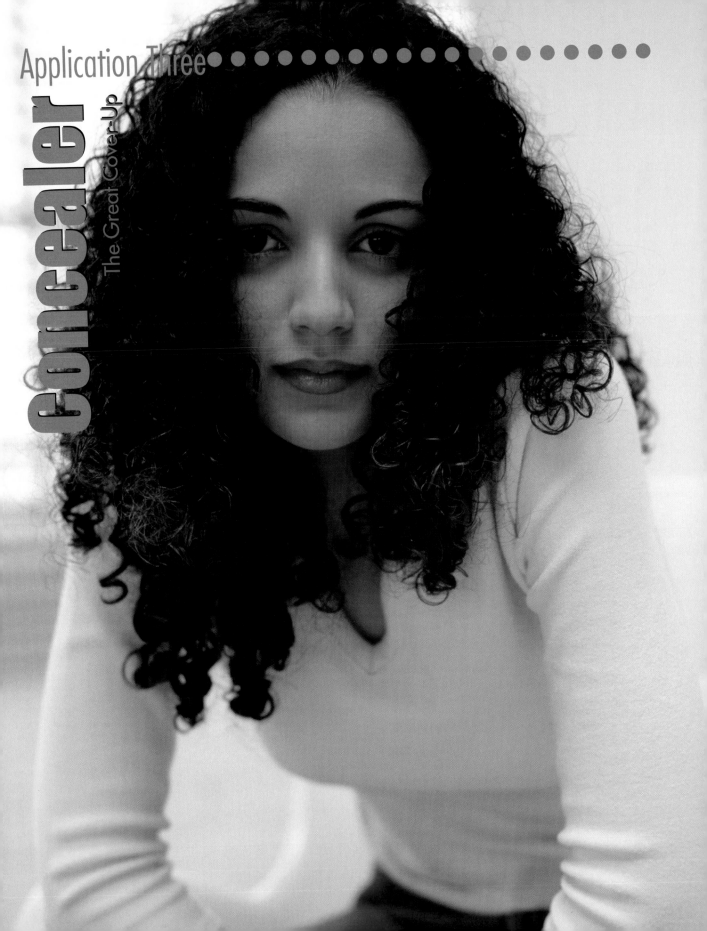

Concealer

The Great Cover-Up

Coneealer teamed with foundation gives your complexion a picture-perfect finish. It's commonly used to cover blemishes and camouflage dark circles under the eyes. However, it can also be used to mask skin discolorations, scars, and birthmarks. Used sparingly, the right concealer gives your skin a flawless finish.

Concealer is the one product you'll want to consider even if you don't normally wear any makeup. Blended with foundation or worn alone, it gives you on-the-spot coverage wherever you need it.

Concealer is the perfect cover-up.

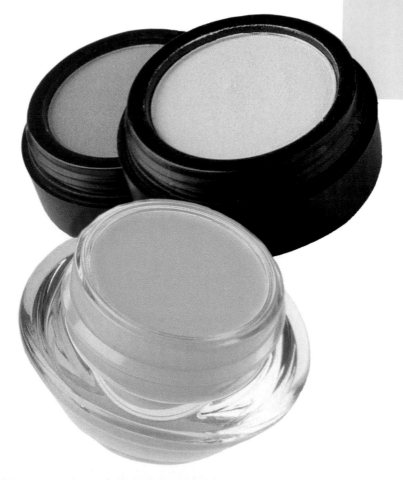

Uncovering the Facts on Cover-Up

Concealer should not be worn as foundation, because it can clog your pores and cause breakouts. Its heavy emollient base is specifically formulated for pimples and hard-to-cover areas under your eyes. Used correctly, concealer makes you look well rested and blemish free.

Check It Out

Choosing a concealer is much easier than choosing foundation. There are only a couple of questions to ask yourself in order to make your selection: What color? and How much coverage?

#1: Color

This step is easy since you've already determined your skin tone when choosing a foundation. Unlike foundations, most concealers only come in three shades. The only thing you have to answer now is whether the color you chose falls into the light, medium, or dark category. Your concealer should be a shade or two lighter than your foundation.

Circle the color that best matches your foundation: Light Medium Dark

#2: Coverage

What type of coverage do you need? If you're using it under your eyes, how dark are the circles? Are you covering blemishes, scratches, scrapes, or scars? Is it for a quick blemish cover-up? Concealers come in several different varieties depending on the use. In the next section I'll introduce what the market has to offer.

Special Note

If you're using concealer alone, without any foundation, you'll want to spend a little more time making your selection. To find the concealer that works best for you, apply a small amount to your skin and gently blend it in. Use your handheld mirror and check the color and coverage in natural daylight. A sheer application of liquid concealer works best, because heavier concealers will leave your face looking spotted.

The Answer Is

Even though the color choices are minimal when choosing concealer, there are many varieties to consider. Allow me to uncover some of the mystery about cover-ups.

Liquid: (light coverage) Liquid concealer is found in a wand or tube. It gives subtle sheer coverage and blends easily. However, unless you set it with translucent powder, it wears off easily.

Cream: (medium coverage) Cream concealer comes in compact and tube form. It's nontransparent and gives good coverage with or without powder.

Solid Stick: (full coverage) Stick concealers offer full coverage for the most difficult skin problems. However, they can be too heavy or greasy depending on the formula you choose.

Medicated: There are a variety of acne treatment concealers on the market. These are usually found where acne medications are shelved.

Beauty Bonus

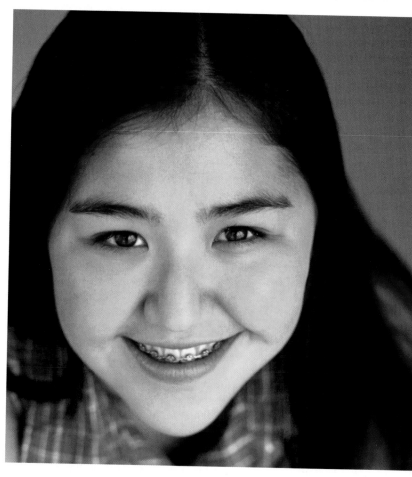

Like foundations, concealers contain extra ingredients that benefit your skin:

Oil-free/Lanolin-free—This product contains little to no oily emollients. It works great on oily acne prone skin, especially when covering blemishes.

Fragrance-free—These products contain no artificial fragrances that can trigger allergies.

Corrective—Yellow cover-up is used under foundation to cancel out the purplish discolorations like circles under your eyes.

Tammy's Tip: For long-lasting lip color, apply concealer to your lips before adding lipstick.

Green cover-up is used to cancel out red discoloration like that associated with blemishes, scars, and broken capillaries.

Pro-Retinol A—This formula helps smooth and soften the appearance of fine lines and wrinkles.

Vitamin E—This featured ingredient also smoothes and softens the appearance of lines and wrinkles.

Benzoyl Peroxide—This medicated ingredient is used to dry skin and heal blemishes.

SPF (Sun Protection Factor)—Concealers that contain an SPF of 15 or higher combat the negative effects of the sun's harmful rays.

Waterproof—Waterproof concealer contains waxy emollients that won't wear off in water.

How It Applies

Apply concealer by itself or after you've put on your foundation. Follow these simple instructions to apply foolproof concealer every time.

Dark Circles under Eyes—Using your ring finger, gently dab a small amount of concealer under your eye. Gently pat and blend with a makeup sponge.

Blemishes—Treat with a medicated blemish cream. Let dry for 3–5 minutes. Using your ring finger, gently dab a small amount on the pimple. Lightly pat on and around the area to blend into your skin.

Scratches or Scars—Use your ring finger to gently dab concealer on the affected area. Let dry 1–2 minutes. Use your makeup sponge to blend. Dust lightly with translucent powder.

Eye Shadow Base—To brighten your eyes and give your eye shadow longevity, apply a small amount of concealer to your eyelid. Blend it from the base of your lash to the base of your brow. Don't use too much, or you'll end up with raccoon eyes! Allow it to set 1 minute and then apply your makeup.

Lip Color Base—Use your ring finger to gently smooth on a sheer application of concealer before you apply your lip color. This will keep your lip color looking fresh.

Putting It to the Test

When you apply a little know-how with your concealer, your face will look virtually flawless. Whether or not you use additional makeup, you'll cover up the bad as you uncover the beautiful.

Use the form on the next page to measure the success of the concealers you try on. Once you have found a perfect match, write the product information in the blanks provided. Cosmetic companies change the names (especially the color names) and packaging of their products quite frequently to keep up with changing trends, but if you know the old product information the company can help you match it to the new products available.

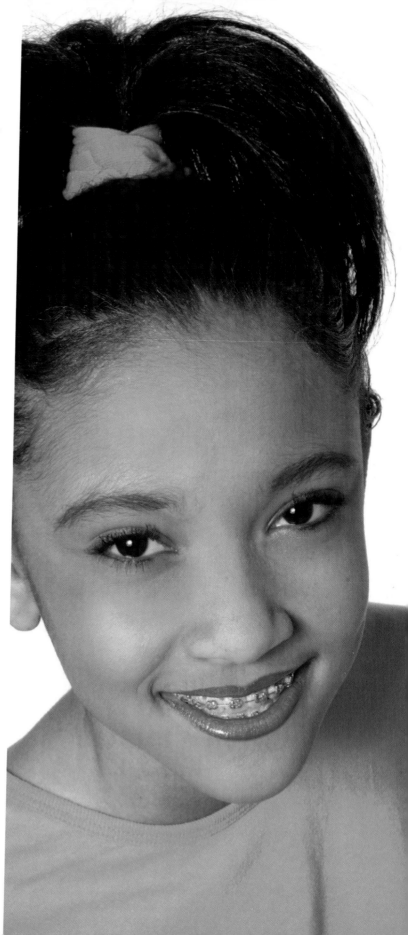

Finding My Concealer

Date:_____

What color best matches your foundation?   Light   Medium   Dark

How much coverage will you need?   Light   Medium   Dark

In the spaces below write down the name of the product and the color you are testing. Determine if it matches your skin tone and sufficiently covers the texture of your skin.

1. Product name:

    Color:

    Does it match your skin tone/foundation?   YES / NO

    Is it the right amount of coverage?   YES / NO

2. Product name:

    Color:

    Does it match your skin tone/foundation?   YES / NO

    Is it the right amount of coverage?   YES / NO

3. Product name:

    Color:

    Does it match your skin tone/foundation?   YES / NO

    Is it the right amount of coverage?   YES / NO

4. Product name:

    Color:

    Does it match your skin tone/foundation?   YES / NO

    Is it the right amount of coverage?   YES / NO

5. Product name:

    Color:

    Does it match your skin tone/foundation?   YES / NO

    Is it the right amount of coverage?   YES / NO

My Perfect Match

Product Name:

Color:

Manufacturer's Name:

The key to flawless skin is uncovered with concealer.

The answer to fault-free skin is found in a tube of concealer. Dark circles under the eyes, blemishes, scars—all seem to vanish with just a tiny amount of this wonder product. Wouldn't it be great if there was a miraculous way to cover up life's blemishes as well? Guess what? There is. It's the blood of Jesus.

In application one we looked at cleansing—the forgiveness of sins by believing in Jesus. Once you trusted in him you became a Christian. Now that you're a Christian, you look at sin from a whole new perspective. It no longer separates you from eternity with God, but it hinders your relationship with him.

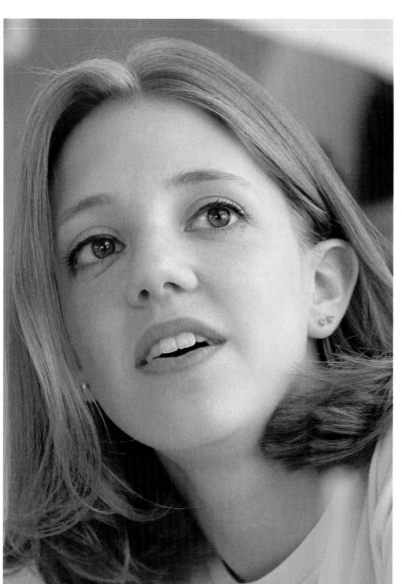

The blood of Jesus is the perfect cover-up.

Speeding, yes speeding! I've struggled with that particular sin ever since I got my driver's license. I usually travel only five or ten miles over the speed limit, going with the flow of traffic. Since everyone else is doing it, does that make it wrong?

See what I mean? I've been at it so long, it's become second nature—my sinful nature, that is. When I'm speeding in my car, the Holy Spirit is right there with me, hurt and saddened that I'm breaking the law and breaking my fellowship with God. God in his perfection cannot be a party to sin.

By the way, sin has consequences and in my case it's known as a speeding ticket. God's used that little slip of paper as a friendly reminder to me that when I'm on the road, I need to slow down!

What happens when you hurt a friend, even when it's unintentional? Hopefully, you apologize and ask forgiveness. Through this your friendship grows and deepens. It's a lesson in integrity and humility. This same example applies to your relationship with Christ. When you mess up, you need to confess and ask forgiveness.

The next few pages will show you how to uncover the truth about sin in the Christian life. Though we've been concealed in Jesus' blood, we still need to reveal our screw-ups. We all mess up, and what's been done can't be undone, but we can still receive forgiveness.

Uncovering the Facts on Cover-Up

We humans never stop sinning, not even as Christians! It's not that we don't want to, but it's hard, almost impossible at times. So the most important question is, what happens when we sin after we've accepted Christ?

First, you need to know that you *never* lose the relationship you have with God the Father. You keep that eternal security as his child no matter what you do. Once you've believed in his son Jesus there's not a sin big enough to sever those ties. It's like the connection you have with your parents: You might make them angry and bruise your relationship with them, but they'll always be your blood parents. It's the same way with God. Your sin might get in the way of your relationship with him, but you'll be his daughter forever because you were adopted by Jesus' blood.

So back to the original question, what happens to Christians when we sin?

Check It Out

Ephesians 4:30—And do not grieve the Holy Spirit of God, with whom you were sealed for the day of redemption.

According to the Bible we break God's heart when we sin. His love for us doesn't change, but our nearness to him does. He doesn't move away from us; we move away from him. God's always the same; it's we who compromise the relationship through our wrongdoing. In fact, the longer we participate in sin, the farther away from God we move. We can get so wrapped up in sinning that we forget we're even doing it.

The Answer Is

There are three steps to uncovering and confessing your sin so you can grow closer to God. Just like the relationship you have with your best friend, talking to one another is the key to growing closer. Your relationship with God is similar, except that he actually dwells in your heart and soul. In order to keep the arteries of communication open with God, you must practice CPR: Confess, Praise, Repent.

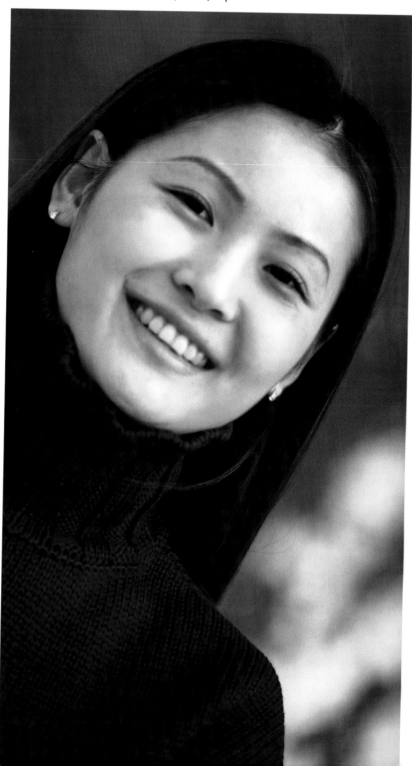

Time Out with Tammy—

In high school I had several best friends. We did everything together until one of them got a girlfriend. Once Roger started dating he stopped hanging out with us, and that made us mad. We started making fun of his girlfriend, Rachel, and even teased him about her. One night, however, we took it too far and hurt Roger's feelings. It was at that point that I realized what we were doing was wrong, and I asked God and Roger to forgive me. Then I went to the rest of the group and talked to them too. We made a pact not to make fun of Rachel again. We held each other accountable to do the right thing. In fact, we even asked Rachel to join our clan, and when we did, we discovered we liked her too!

Tammy's Tip
Nothing is concealed from the eyes of God.

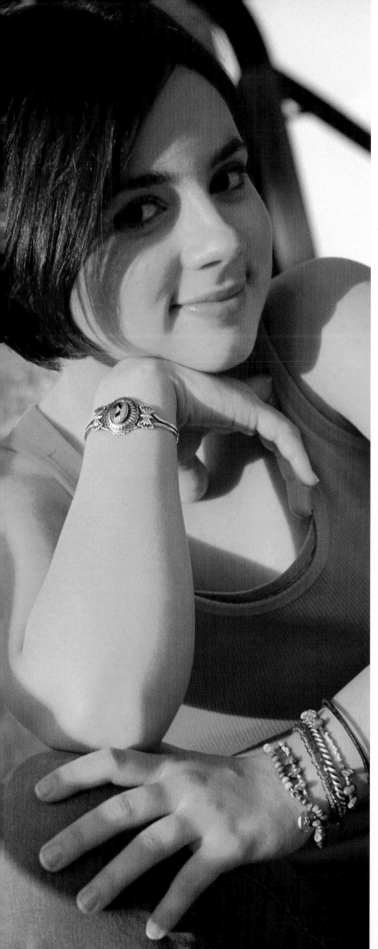

#1: Confess

Confess your sins to God. Be honest and humble—he already knows what you did. Even in the most difficult situations he's waiting to forgive you.

Proverbs 28:13—He who conceals his sins does not prosper, but whoever confesses and renounces them finds mercy.

#2: Praise

Praise God for bringing sins to your attention that need forgiveness, and then praise him for forgiving you.

2 Timothy 4:18—The Lord will rescue me from every evil attack and will bring me safely to his heavenly kingdom. To him be glory for ever and ever. Amen.

#3: Repent

Repent from your sin. Do a 180-degree turn and run! If it's something you struggle with on a continual basis, ask God to help you overcome it.

Revelation 3:19—Be earnest, and repent.

Beauty Bonus

If you're struggling with sin that you can't seem to master on your own, ask your friends for help. Friends can be a great source of accountability.

How It Applies

Any relationship that's worth having requires work to maintain. A relationship with God is the best one you can have, but it's the greatest risk. Satan will do anything in his power to break it off, even though he can never end it. He has only one goal in mind, and that is to damage your relationship with God. If he can successfully entice you to sin, then he can use that sin against you and damage your witness for God.

Be smart about Satan's tricks. Don't put yourself in a situation where you'll be tempted to sin. But remember, if you do make a mistake, God is right there waiting to forgive you. All you have to do is ask. Sin will cover up who you are in Christ, unless you uncover it with confession, praise, and repentance.

Putting It to the Test

Concealer allows you to give flawed skin the look of perfection, just as the blood of Jesus covers our many sins, making us perfect before God. Concealer to the skin is what cover-up, Jesus' blood, is to the soul. So make the effort to uncover your sins and give your sinful heart some CPR.

Confess, Praise, Repent. Use it. Apply it. You'll be amazed at what a difference it makes in your spiritual life.

Beauty Secret #3: Cover-up uncovers the "Super Model" in you.

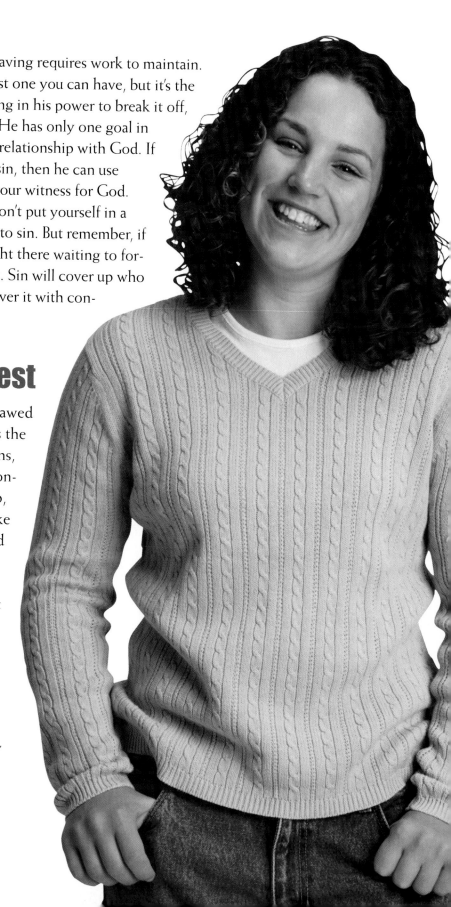

Blush

The Bold and the Beautiful

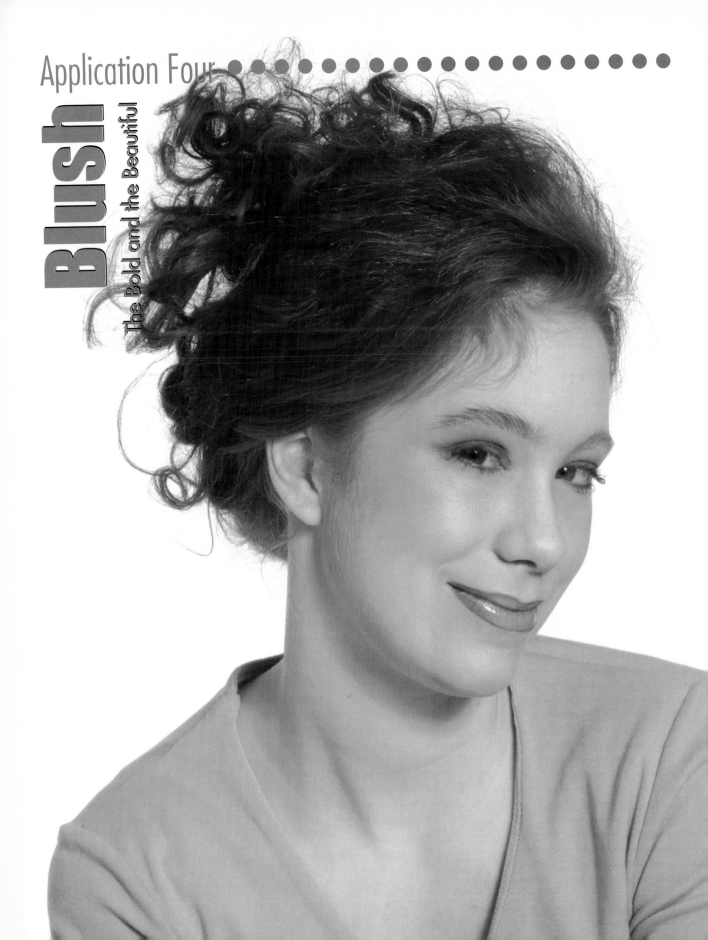

Before there was the convenience of blusher or rouge, girls tortured themselves by pinching themselves up and down their cheekbones to achieve just the right amount of blushing color. Bashfulness, though not always sincere, was an alluring quality that attracted gentlemen callers. This was during a time when guys liked to be the pursuers and not the pursued. My, how times have changed! Now we get all gussied up, boldly brush on the blush, and aggressively go after whatever we want. I'm not just talking about guys; I'm talking about anything we're the least bit interested in.

Aren't you glad we no longer live in a time where we have to pinch our cheeks until they're red and swollen to achieve a healthy-looking glow? However, we do tend to torment ourselves by wasting time and money on wrong blushers. In this application you'll learn how to avoid costly mistakes and expertly buy and apply the perfect blush for your skin.

Blush emphasizes your cheekbones with an accent of color.

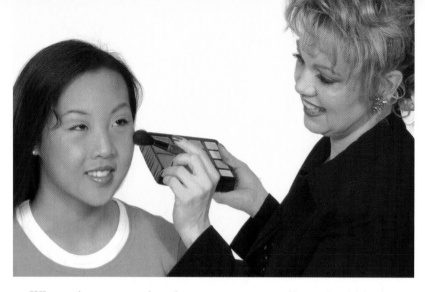

Worn alone or with other cosmetics, well-applied blusher serves two general purposes. It gives the palest of skin a fresh healthy glow, and it also gives you well-defined supermodel cheekbones.

The Blushing Facts

Buying the right blush is relatively easy. There are really only two questions you have to ask yourself. What color will look best with my skin tone? And what kind do I want to wear?

Check It Out

#1: Color

Blush comes in a variety of colors: everything from tints of pink, to shades of peach and plum. The color you choose depends on your color palette. Is your skin light-, medium-, or dark-complexioned, and is your hair *naturally* blonde, red (including strawberry blonde to russet browns), brown, black, or gray?

Circle the color that best matches your skin tone: LIGHT   MEDIUM   DARK

Circle your *natural* hair color:

BLONDE   RED (strawberry blonde/russet browns)   BROWN   BLACK   GRAY

Using the chart on the next page, cross-reference your skin tone and hair color to locate the best colors for you to sample. You may want to experiment with more than one color for the perfect look. Remember that color names continually change with the trends. You'll see everything on the market from orange sherbet (peach), wild raspberry (pink), to toasted almond (brown).

	Light/Fair	Medium	Dark
Blonde	Light to medium tints of pink, mauve, or rose colors	Medium shades of pink, mauve, rose, or plum colors	Medium to dark shades of mauve, plum, wine, or bronzy brown tones
Red (strawberry blonde to russet browns)	Light to medium tints of peach, coral, or apricot colors	Medium shades of peach, coral, or apricot colors	Medium to dark shades of coral, apricot, or warm nutmeg tones
Brown	Light to medium shades of peachy pink (you may have to buy one in each color)	Medium shades of peachy mauve (you may have to buy one in each color)	Medium to dark shades of mocha plum or warm bark tones
Black	Light to medium tints of pink, mauve, or rose colors	Medium shades of pink, mauve, rose, or plum colors	Medium to dark shades of mauve, plum, wine, or bronzy brown tones
Gray	Light to medium tints of pink, mauve, or rose colors	Medium shades of pink, mauve, rose, or plum colors	Medium to dark shades of mauve, plum, wine, or bronzy brown tones

Have fun and experiment with an array of colors until you find one or two that work for you!

#2: Kind

There are basically five types of blush or rouge to choose from: powder, cream, liquid, gel, or stick. You'll want to use the consistency that blends most easily into your skin, giving you a natural healthy-looking glow.

The Answer Is

So we never get bored buying them, blushers are packaged and repackaged in an assortment of cutesy compacts, tubes, wands, and sticks. To help you avoid packaging gimmicks, I've done your product homework for you.

Tammy's Tip
In a pinch, substitute lipstick for blush.

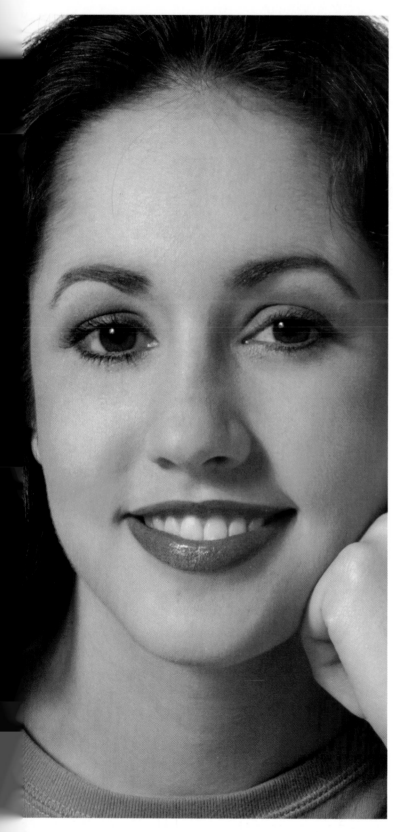

Powder—Powder blush blends well on all skin types and comes in the largest selection of colors. It can be purchased in dual or multicolored compacts for extra color flexibility and contouring.

Cream—Cream blusher or rouge can contain additives such as SPF 10 and vitamins C and E. It blends nicely on dry and mature skin and doesn't cake in fine lines.

Liquid—Liquid blush offers added ingredients such as SPF 10, vitamins C and E, and bronzing crystal complex (face illuminator). It can be difficult to apply evenly and often ends up looking blotchy. It can also stain clothing.

Gel—Gels are tricky to rub into the skin without streaking. They too can stain clothing.

Stick—Sticks come in oil-free, water-based, and emollient rich formulas. They go on creamy, blend easily, and provide sheer translucent color to most skin types. However, they can look blotchy.

Beauty Bonus

There are an assortment of formulated features that cosmetic manufacturers offer to improve the quality of the product and the condition of your skin. Here are a few of the most recent blush additives.

Oil-free/Water-based—This product contains little to no oily emollients. It works well on oily acne-prone skin.

Fragrance-free—These products contain no artificial fragrances that can trigger allergies.

Vitamins E and C—This vitamin combination smoothes and softens the appearance of fine lines and wrinkles.

SPF (Sun Protection Factor)—Blushers that contain a SPF of 15 or higher combat the negative effects of the sun's harmful rays.

How It Applies

Applying blush is relatively easy if you follow a few simple guidelines.

Finding Your Cheekbones—Smile to find the apples of your cheeks. This is where you naturally blush.

Basic Application—Using a blush brush (a soft medium-sized brush with rounded bristles) lightly sweep blush across your cheekbone in an upward and outward stroke. Start from the middle of your eye, brushing towards your hairline but not into your hairline. Only apply a little at a time, repeating this process as necessary. Applying too little blush is far better than too much!

Blending—Use the wide base of a makeup sponge to gently blend your blush, softening the edges. I do this step twice to make sure there is absolutely no blush line.

Contouring—Give your cheekbones a well-shaped lift by contouring two colors of blush together. Apply the darker of the two shades on the upper edge of your cheekbone by following the basic application directions. Next use the lighter tint, contouring just beneath the darker color. Now gently sweep your brush upwards and outwards, blending the two colors. Finally, follow the blending directions to blend color into your skin.

Putting It to the Test

When you artfully apply blusher to your cheekbones, you give your face illuminating color that creates an instant face-lift. You'll look healthy and refreshed even if you stayed up all night.

Some experts recommend applying your eye makeup first so you don't put on too much blush, and others recommend applying blush

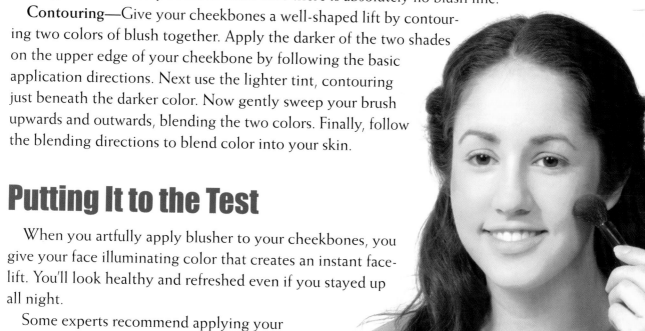

Tammy's Tip • • • • • • • • • • • • For a softer look, dip your blush brush into loose powder before you dip it into your blusher.

Finding My Blusher

Date: _____

What is your skin tone?   Light   Medium   Dark

What are your best colors? Using the chart on page 61, write down the colors that would be best for you to sample.

In the spaces below write down the name of the product and the color you are testing. Determine if it matches your skin tone and blends easily.

1. Product name: Color:

   Does it match your skin tone?   **YES / NO**

   Does it blend easily?   **YES / NO**

2. Product name: Color:

   Does it match your skin tone?   **YES / NO**

   Does it blend easily?   **YES / NO**

3. Product name: Color:

   Does it match your skin tone?   **YES / NO**

   Does it blend easily?   **YES / NO**

My Perfect Match

Product Name: Color:

Manufacturer's Name:

first so you don't overdo your eyes. I say either way you do it, make sure you don't get carried away. You want people to notice you, not your makeup.

Use the form above to measure the success of the blushers you sample. Once you have found a perfect match, write the product information in the blanks provided. Cosmetic companies change the names (especially color names) and packaging of their products quite frequently to keep up with changing trends, but if you know the old product information the company can help you match it to the new products available.

Tammy's Tip
The goal is to use makeup without looking made up.

The key to well-defined cheekbones is a blushing glow.

The purpose of blush is to give you a healthy glow without overdoing it. Once applied, you want it to look natural. The goal here is to wear makeup without looking all made up. The same is true in our Christian lives. As the bride of Christ, we want to be witnesses for him—what bride doesn't like to brag about her husband? But we don't want to turn people off by overdoing it. The goal is to be sold out for Christ without becoming a pushy salesperson.

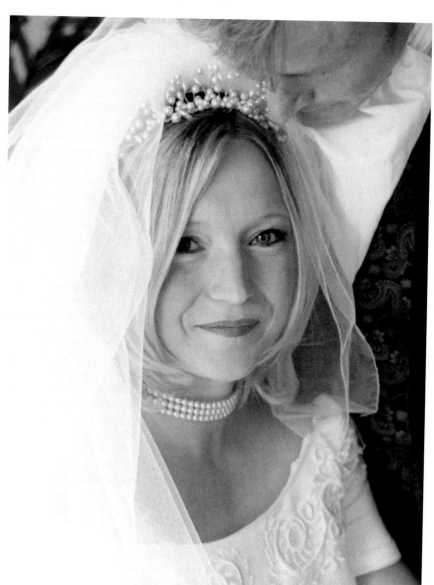

Christians don't need to blush when they live boldly by example.

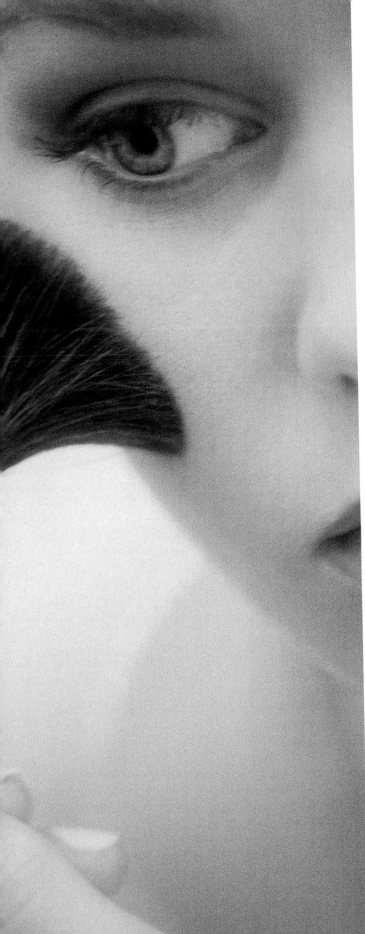

It's often said that after you've been married to someone for a while you start acting and looking alike. This is especially true for Christians. As brides of Christ, we should become more Christ-like everyday. People see God living in you by you living for God.

Jackie's dad didn't know the Lord. No matter how many times she asked him to go to church, he wouldn't go. But even though Jackie had asked Christ into her life, she never changed her behavior. She ignored her dad all week but wanted him to listen to her on Sunday. One evening at youth group the topic was "Changed Heart, Changed Life." Jackie realized her conduct hadn't been what it should be. She went home that evening and apologized to her dad for her disobedience and promised to do better. Over the next few weeks, Jackie's dad noticed a significant change in his daughter. The next time she invited him to church, he went. When Jackie finally walked the talk, her dad listened, and now he knows the Lord too!

The Blushing Facts

You can do more damage than good if you say one thing and do another. Talk is cheap when there are no actions to follow it up. If you believe something, live it out, and you'll make others want to be believers too! Your actions will light the way to salvation in Christ.

Matthew 5:14–16—"You are the light of the world. A city on a hill cannot be hidden. Neither do people light a lamp and put it under a bowl. Instead they put it on its stand, and it gives light to everyone in the house. In the same way, let your light shine before men, that they may see your good deeds and praise your Father in heaven."

One night my family and I were traveling across the desert, and we could see a great glow of lights in the distance. We were tired and hungry and relieved to know we'd be in a town soon. We drove on with little patience and great anticipation for many miles before we finally got there. From a far off distance, that tiny desert town gave off a tremendous amount of light that could be seen in the darkness of the desert.

This was only a small town, not even on a hill, and yet the lights led us on.

"You are the light of the world. A city on a hill cannot be hidden."

Jesus used this word picture to illustrate how Christians are like city lights—blinking from the top of a hill and surrounded by the darkness of sin.

Your life is that light. When kids see how you act at school, you'll stand out like a neon sign. Even if you never say a word, they'll notice something different about you just by your behavior.

People will notice that you're not perfect and that you sin, but what they'll notice even more is that when you mess up you don't give up. Your light might flicker, but it will never go out.

"Neither do people light a lamp and put it under a bowl. Instead they put it on its stand, and it gives light to everyone in the house. In the same way, let your light shine before men, that they may see your good deeds and praise your Father in heaven."

In other words don't hide the fact that you're a Christian. That's all there is to it. You don't have to shout it from the

Time-Out
with Tammy—

We're often unaware that anyone is watching us unless it's brought to our attention. I once met a girl who was in serious trouble; she was huffing gas. She had already gone through rehab and relapsed. She didn't like what she was doing, but she didn't know how to stop. She felt alone and hopeless when she came to me for help. She said she knew I was a Christian by the way I acted, and she wanted to know if God could help her stop hurting herself. I was able to share Jesus with her because she saw Christ living in me. It was nothing I said, just the way I behaved. And the remarkable thing is, she came to me. I didn't have to go looking for her.

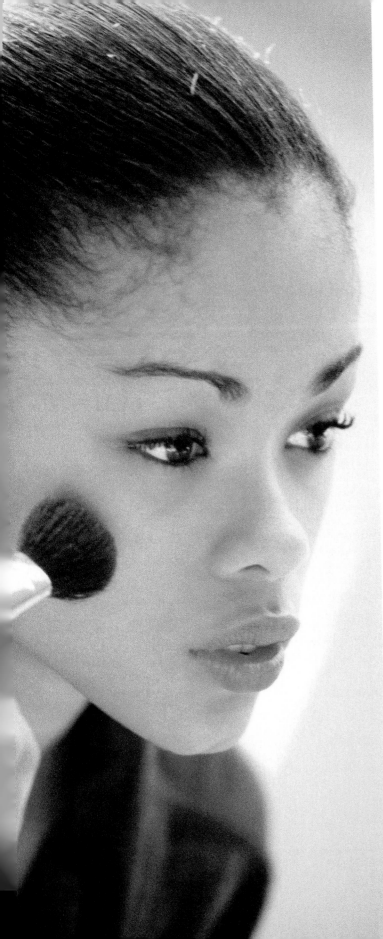

rooftop of your school; just live it. When we live our daily lives according to what the Bible says, others will notice Christ living in us.

Check It Out

It's difficult to be a teenager and a testimony all at one time. I know firsthand how hard it is to feel scrutinized under the forces of peer pressure. Satan delights in embarrassing you, and he sends people to harass you for doing the right thing. He wants to make you feel bad enough that you'll forget about living for Christ and ruin your testimony. Think of it this way: If you weren't living the right way, Satan wouldn't try so hard to make you feel so wrong.

The Answer Is

Walking the walk is key to your testimony. Sure, talking the talk is important. But if you're saying one thing and doing another, no one is going to listen. *L.I.V.E.* your life according to God's purpose and everyone will hear you loud and clear.

Listen to yourself. Are you a nice person to talk to or are you judgmental and demeaning to those who are not like you? What kind of language do you use? Cursing will wreck your testimony.

Identify your weaknesses and avoid them. For example, if going to parties is going to tempt you to drink alcohol, then *don't go to parties!*

Value your relationship with Christ. Keep your foundation strong through the Word, prayer, church, and Christian friendships.

Express your faith in what you do and don't do, how you act, and what you wear. That's right—even your clothes can testify.

Tammy's Tip • • • • • • • • •
Always remember actions speak louder than words.

Beauty Bonus

There will be times when you mess up, do something you shouldn't, and blow your testimony. What happens then? Admit your guilt to God, pick yourself up, brush yourself off, and carry on. To err is human, but to acknowledge your mistakes and humbly apologize is a true witness to God's grace.

How It Applies

Blush gives you a healthy-looking glow on the outside. Jesus gives you a radiance that glows from the inside out. Remember, this childhood song, and let your light shine!

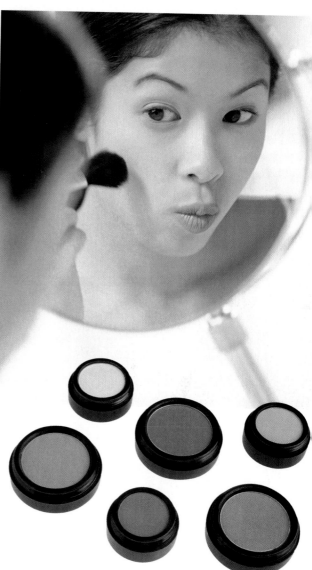

This Little Light of Mine

This little light of mine, I'm gonna let it shine.
This little light of mine, I'm gonna let it shine.
This little light of mine, I'm gonna let it shine.
Let it shine, let it shine, let it shine.

Hide it under a bushel? NO! I'm gonna let it shine.
Hide it under a bushel? NO! I'm gonna let it shine.
Hide it under a bushel? NO! I'm gonna let it shine.
Let it shine, let it shine, let it shine.

Won't let Satan blow it out. I'm gonna let it shine.
Won't let Satan blow it out. I'm gonna let it shine.
Won't let Satan blow it out. I'm gonna let it shine.
Let it shine, let it shine, let it shine.

Putting It to the Test

Your actions are your greatest witnessing tool. Don't blush over your decision to follow Christ, but be bold in your love for him. Give it a try. Make the change today.

Beauty Secret #4: A blushing glow boldly lights up the "Super Model" in you.

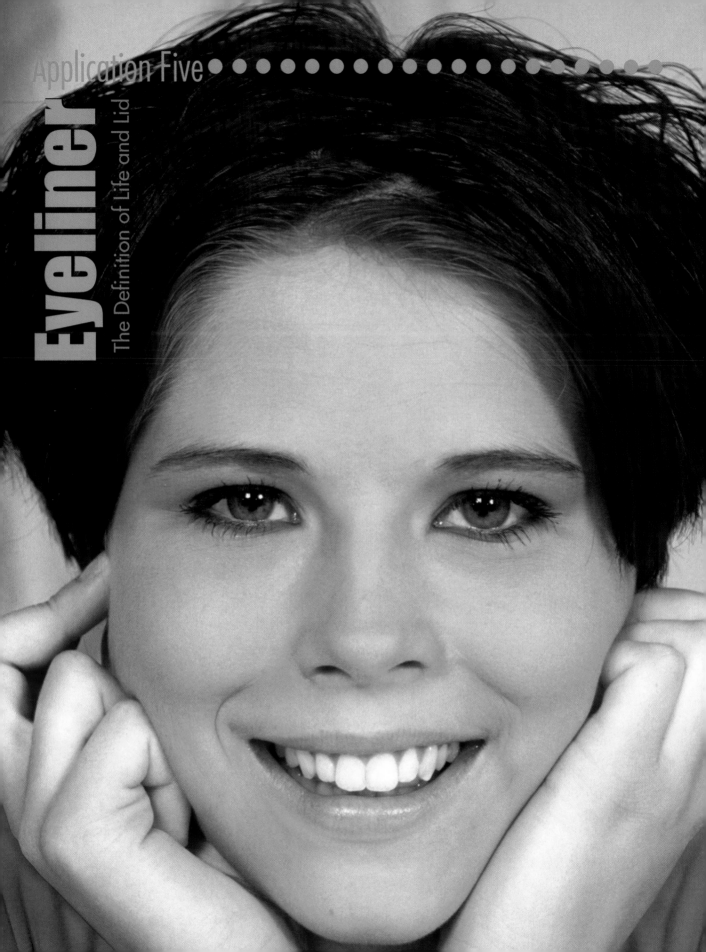

Eyeliner
The Definition of Life and Lid

Eyeliner is used to give pronounced depth and definition to the eyes. When applied well, it opens narrow eyes, broadens close-set eyes, and tapers wide, round eyes, for an eye-catching effect. It's similar to coloring in a coloring book. You can color the picture and it looks nice, but if you outline the picture, it pops off the page at you. Eyeliner is an added touch that sets you apart from the amateurs.

Effective eyeliner is much more than drawing circles around your lash line. It should be used to perfect the contour of your eyes. I'm going to give you the eyeliner details you need to avoid looking like an amateur and start looking like a professional.

Eyeliner gives definition to the shape of your eyes.

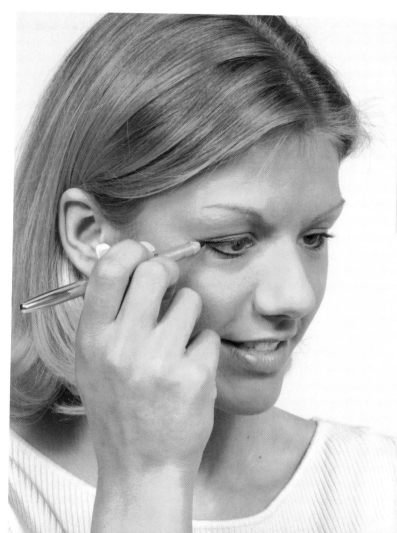

71

Outlined Facts on Lids

There are minimal choices when it comes to purchasing eyeliner. The real benefit comes when you apply it. To help you narrow down your choices, let's first take a look at the kind of application you're going to need by determining the shape of your eyes.

Check It Out

Do you have close-set eyes?

The spacing between your eyes is minimal. Your objective is to emphasize the outer corners of your eyes.

Do you have wide-set eyes?

You have a broad space between your eyes creating the need to emphasize the inner corners of your eyes.

Do you have deep-set eyes?

Your eyes appear sunken and hollow. Your goal is to bring them to the surface by minimizing the use of eyeliner.

Do you have small narrow eyes?

Small eyes can be opened up to look larger by concentrating liner on the outer corners of your eyes.

Do you have large round eyes?

Extending your liner beyond the outer edge of your eyes can visually lengthen large round eyes.

What if your eyes are none of the above?

If your eyes don't fall into any of the other categories, then congratulations—you have eyes that require no special attention to any given area.

Check It Out

Now that you know what you need to accomplish, let's determine how you're going to achieve it.

#1: Kind

There are three basic forms of eyeliner: liquid, pencil, or wet/dry shadows. Since each of them wears about the same, pick the one that's easiest for you to apply.

#2: Color

Though the kinds of eyeliner are limited, some are offered in an array of colors. Liquid eyeliners come in basic tones like brown, black, or black/brown. However, pencils and wet/dry shadows are offered in a range of colors, everything from espresso brown to emerald green.

The Answer Is

The key to professional-looking eyeliner is finding one that is easy for you to apply. My personal favorite is eyeliner pencil because it gives me absolute and complete control.

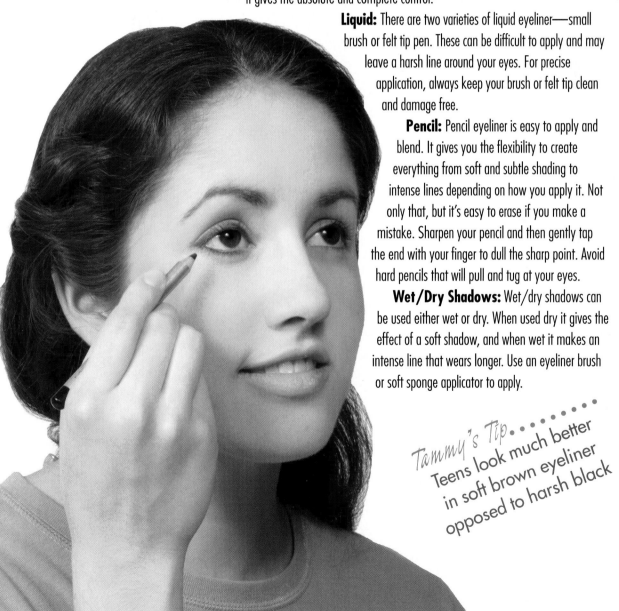

Liquid: There are two varieties of liquid eyeliner—small brush or felt tip pen. These can be difficult to apply and may leave a harsh line around your eyes. For precise application, always keep your brush or felt tip clean and damage free.

Pencil: Pencil eyeliner is easy to apply and blend. It gives you the flexibility to create everything from soft and subtle shading to intense lines depending on how you apply it. Not only that, but it's easy to erase if you make a mistake. Sharpen your pencil and then gently tap the end with your finger to dull the sharp point. Avoid hard pencils that will pull and tug at your eyes.

Wet/Dry Shadows: Wet/dry shadows can be used either wet or dry. When used dry it gives the effect of a soft shadow, and when wet it makes an intense line that wears longer. Use an eyeliner brush or soft sponge applicator to apply.

Tammy's Tip • • • • • • • • •
Teens look much better in soft brown eyeliner opposed to harsh black

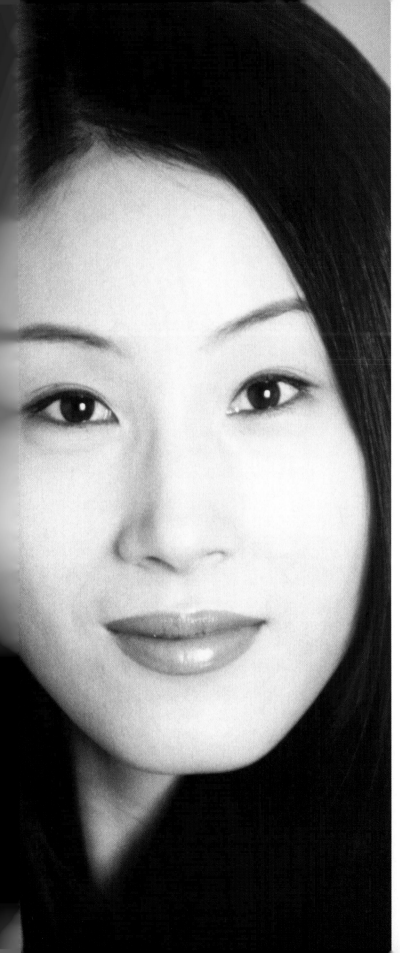

Beauty Bonus

When it comes to eye makeup, it's okay to be stingy. I know you've always been taught to share, but this rule doesn't apply to products that come in contact with the eyes. The eye area is highly sensitive, and sharing eye products such as liners, shadows, or mascara can easily lead to infections.

How It Applies

Once you get the hang of it, eyeliner is fairly easy to apply. It just takes a little know-how. Follow the advice below and you'll be a pro in no time.

Determine Eye Type. Your eyeliner will only be successful if it is applied according to the type of eyes you have. (Refer to page 72.)

Basic Application. Locate the type of eyes you have and then follow the directions.

Close-set Eyes—Line both your upper and lower lids from the center of your eyelid outward. Gently blend.

Wide-set Eyes—Starting in the corner of your eye, line both the upper and lower lids two-thirds of the way across. Then gently blend to the outer edge.

Deep-set Eyes—Start one-fourth of the way from the inner

Tammy's Tip
When using a pencil, start from the outside of your eye and work your way in to avoid stretching the skin around the eye area.

corner of your eye and work toward the outer edge. Apply a fine line at the base of both your upper and lower lashes and blend.

Small Narrow Eyes—Line both your upper and lower lids from the center of your eyelid out. Extend the line from the outer edge upward and outward and blend.

Large Round Eyes—Start at the inner corner of your upper eyelid and work toward the outer edge, extending the line outward and upward. Line only the outer corner beneath your eye, blending it upward and outward also.

None of the Above—Start at the inner corner of your eye and apply outward and slightly upward once you reach the outer edge. Follow this process on the upper and lower base of your lashes.

Blending. Use the narrow edge of a makeup sponge to gently blend or smudge your liner. It also works great on erasing mistakes.

Keep it on. Set your eyeliner and avoid smearing by applying a light natural shadow lightly over the top. For the same result, try dipping your shadow brush in translucent powder, tapping off the excess, and gently sweeping it over your liner.

Layering. Another thing you might try for fun is wearing two colors of eyeliner. For example, apply brown liner the way you normally would and then apply a pretty sapphire blue over the top for a two-tone effect.

A makeup artist in Hollywood once told me that the key to successful eyeliner is giving your eyes exact balance. The space you create between your eyes should equal the width of one of your eyes.

Tammy's Tip . . . . *Avoid drawing skimpy incomplete lines with your eyeliner. If you do miss a spot, be sure to fill it in.*

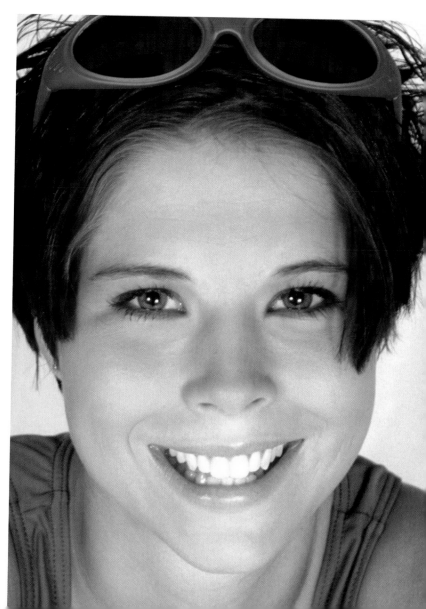

Putting It to the Test

Use the following form to measure the success of the eyeliners you sample. Once you have found one that's easy to apply, practice, practice, practice. Experiment with different colors and have fun with it.

Finding My Eyeliner

Date:_____

What type of eyes do you have?

Close-set   Wide-set   Deep-set   Small/Narrow   Large/Round

None of the Above

Colors of eyeliners I want to try:

In the spaces below write down the type of product and the color you are testing.

Determine how easy it is to apply.

1. Product name:

   Color:

   How easy is it to apply?   EASY   NOT SO EASY   DIFFICULT

   Does it blend easily?   YES/NO

2. Product name:

   Color:

   How easy is it to apply?   EASY   NOT SO EASY   DIFFICULT

   Does it blend easily?   YES/NO

3. Product name:

   Color:

   How easy is it to apply?   EASY   NOT SO EASY   DIFFICULT

   Does it blend easily?   YES/NO

My Perfect Match

Product Name:

Color:

Manufacturer's Name:

The key to expressive eyes is outlined in eyeliner.

Eyeliner brings balanced definition to eyes of all shapes and sizes. Eyes that would normally go unnoticed are brought to life by carefully outlining them to reach their fullest potential.

Our lives should be no different. We spend countless hours each week staring in the mirror, perfecting our looks—but when it comes to life, we tend to leave things to "chance." God has a plan for each one of us. And just like our eyeliner, our lives must be outlined with goals so we too can reach our fullest potential.

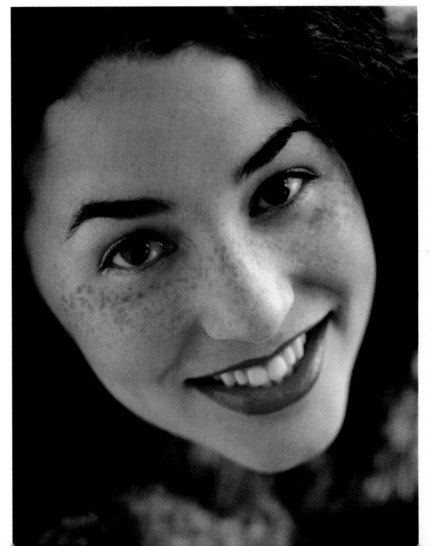

Keeping your eyes in line with God's plan brings definition to life.

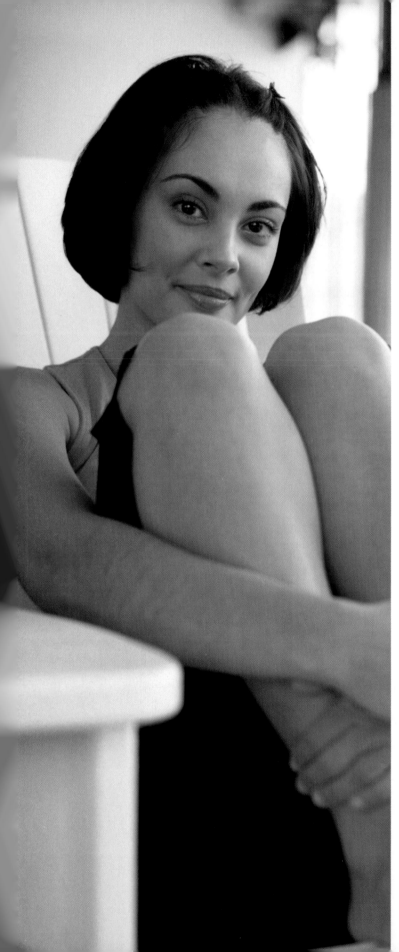

God has a purpose for you. In fact, he had a plan for your life before you were born. Now the only question is, "What is it?" For those of you who have already figured it out, this application will help you stay balanced as you pursue God's goals for your life. And for those of you who are struggling to bring some definition into your lives, this application will show you how to seek God's direction.

Proverbs 3:5–6—Trust in the Lord with all your heart and lean not on your own understanding; in all your ways acknowledge him, and he will make your paths straight.

These are some of my favorite verses. In fact, I love them so much that I've memorized them and have them hanging in my office. Why? I need a constant reminder to trust God's plan instead of trying to do everything my own way. When you read it, it seems simple enough; but reading it and doing it are two different matters.

Following you will find four basic principles. They helped me understand how to practice Proverbs 3:5–6 so I could find my potential through God's direction.

Outlined Facts on Life

Life isn't always easy. And you're at an age where you're making huge decisions with very little experience. The teenage years are the most difficult, demanding, and decisive of any time in your life. Difficult because you're deciding who you are, who your friends are, and how to fit in. Demanding because balancing school, work, family, and friends isn't easy. And decisive because the decisions you make today affect you for the rest of your life. That's where the four principles come in. Having this knowledge will help you deal with everyday life while you're making long-term plans.

Check It Out

I know what you're thinking. You can hardly pick out what you're going to wear tomorrow let alone think about lifelong ambitions! However, it's not as difficult as it sounds if you follow these practical steps:

#1. Love God.
#2. Put others before yourself.
#3. Seek wise counsel.
#4. Be a person of good character.

The Answer Is

#1: Love God

Matthew 22:37—Jesus replied: "'Love the Lord your God with all your heart and with all your soul and with all your mind.'"

God didn't pull any punches on this verse. He covered every area of our lives without question. We are to love him physically with our hearts, spiritually with our souls, and mentally with our minds. Our whole being is to love him first and foremost.

You need to take responsibility for your relationship with God so that you can love him with all your heart, soul, and mind. This kind of love will help you establish your hopes and dreams according to his plan for your life.

Time Out with Tammy—

My husband often refers to 2 Chronicles 34:1—8 when he talks to teens about their relationship with God. It tells about an eight-year-old named Josiah who became king of Judah. Between the ages of eight and fifteen, he automatically did everything he'd seen his father David doing, which included doing what was right in the sight of the Lord. However, at the age of sixteen he started searching for God himself. And by the age of twenty-six, the Bible tells us that he had accepted God for his own.

So how does this apply to you? Simple. Where are you in your God connection? Are you like the eight-year-old Josiah—going to church because your parents make you? Or are you like the sixteen-year-old Josiah who is looking for God? Or do you know and love God on your own like Josiah at twenty-six?

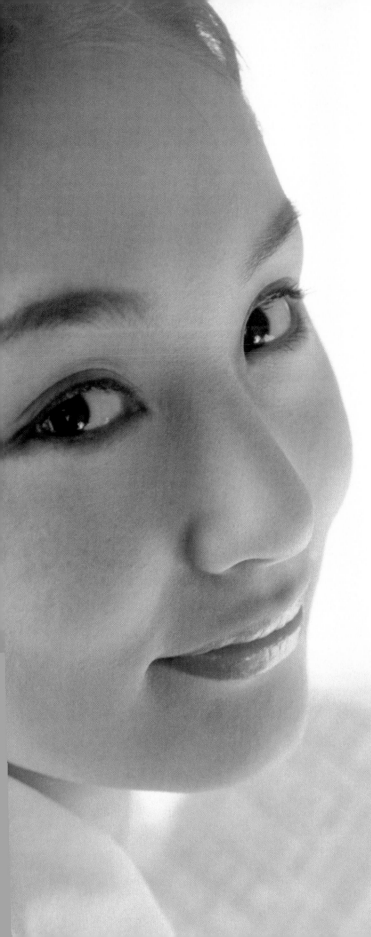

#2: Put others before yourself

Matthew 22:39—"And the second [command-ment] is like it: 'Love your neighbor as yourself.'"

This is a tall order. "Love your neighbor as yourself." We are to treat everyone the way we want to be treated. I'm sure you've heard, "Do unto others as you would have them do unto you." So who qualifies as your neighbor? The people next door? The kids at school? The homeless on the streets? Yes, yes, and yes—your neighbors are anyone you come in contact with. Your neighbors are even your sisters and brothers.

When you love and care for others the way you care for yourself, it will be returned to you many times over. It reminds me of the old saying, "What goes around comes around." I can't think of a greater lifelong achievement than to love and be loved.

#3: Seek wise counsel

Proverbs 15:22—Plans fail for lack of counsel, but with many advisers they succeed.

There are many places you can find answers to your questions. A great place to start is the Bible. The Scriptures are loaded with advice on guys, dating, and sex! But what about those topics you're not so sure about? Like which college to go to or which dress to buy for the prom? Find someone you can trust—a good friend, a teacher, or even your parents. For those of you involved in a youth group, ask your leader for input.

I've found that one of my best counselors is my conscience. Have you ever heard the motto, "Let your conscience be your guide?" More often than not, my gut feeling leads me toward the right choice.

If you talk to any successful person, you will discover they had someone who was instrumental in their success. I could never have completed this book without the support of special friends. Wise counsel will encourage you to realize your dreams and reach your goals.

#4: Be a person of good character.

Titus 2:7–8—In everything set them an example by doing what is good. In your teaching show integrity, seriousness and soundness of speech that cannot be condemned, so that those who oppose you may be ashamed because they have nothing bad to say about us.

Being a person of good moral character is by far the best kind of person you can be.

A person of good character does the right thing even when no one is watching.

The Bible calls us to be honest in *all* we say and do. This includes every area of our lives, whether at home, school, work, or play. Even our enemies should find us faultless.

You'll meet moral opposition every day in one form or another. Whether it's an argument with your parents or the temptation to cheat on your homework, your character will continually be put to the test.

As you pursue goals, do it with high standards of excellence and character. It's easy to go after your dreams with such diligence that you overlook your values and sacrifice moral judgment to get what you want. For example, you want to be a model. Your big break comes along, but it involves modeling lingerie. It's not completely revealing, but it's definitely not modest. What do you do? You'll face tough decisions no matter what career path you choose. Be prepared by keeping your foundation in Christ strong.

Something I do every morning before I step out of bed is say this little prayer: "Lord, please help me do the right thing today." It has made me more aware of what I say and do. Often when I'm faced with a choice I hear those four little words: *Do the right thing.* It's not always easy, but it does trigger my conscience to kick in, which usually helps me make the right choices.

Make "do the right thing" your motto as you live life, outline plans, and establish goals.

Tammy's Tip • • • • • • • •
Say this little prayer before you get out of bed: "Lord, please help me to do the right thing today."

Beauty Bonus

Keep a detailed diary of your hopes and dreams. Write down your short-term and long-term goals and then make plans on how to attain them. It doesn't matter how silly they may seem. Write them down, read them over, and put them in a place where you can see them every day (I keep mine on my makeup mirror). For example:

Short-Term Goals

Do better in math—get tutoring

Go out with Matt—get to know him better first

Buy a new CD—save money

Spend time with God—pray first thing in A.M.

Long-Term Goals

Attend college—prepare for SAT

Become a schoolteacher—become a teacher's aide

Buy a car—save money for car, insurance, tags

Marry a Christian—don't date non-Christians

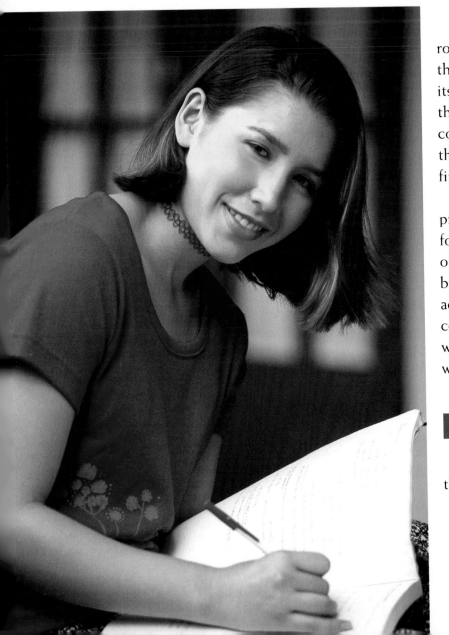

Your goals might even be narrowed down to that day. I write the things I want to accomplish on Post-its. I then go back and prioritize them on a scale of one to five. As I complete them, I peel them off and throw them away. The ones I don't finish, I carry over to the next day.

I've found that keeping a diary and prioritizing daily tasks helps me stay focused on what's important. It not only shows me what I have to do, but it also reminds me of what I've accomplished whenever I feel discouraged. The real key is to do whatever it takes to fulfill your plans with your goals in mind.

How It Applies

Each of us aspires to do something. But without a plan, we're like a person going on a trip with no map; we have a destination in mind but no idea how to get there. We drive around aimlessly, wondering if we're on the right track, and then we come to a roadblock. Life needs a map—a plan for where you want to be today, tomorrow, and ten years from now. And when you meet obstacles, you'll be better prepared to handle them with purpose. Start mapping out your life today.

Putting It to the Test

Take four steps in the right direction. Love God, put others before yourself, seek wise counsel, and be a person of good character. Write these principles, as well as your short-term and long-term goals, down on three-by-five-inch cards and refer to them often. Outlining your life according to God's plan guarantees an excellent future.

Beauty Secret #5: Pencil in, outline, and define the "Super Model" in you.

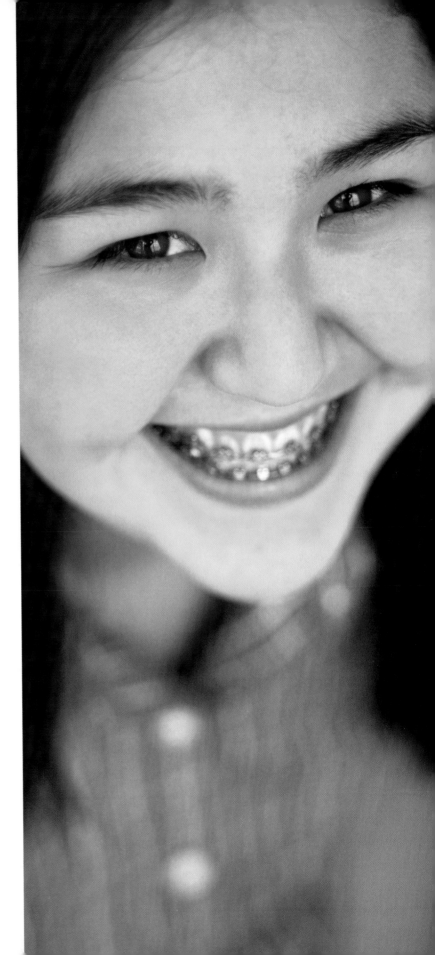

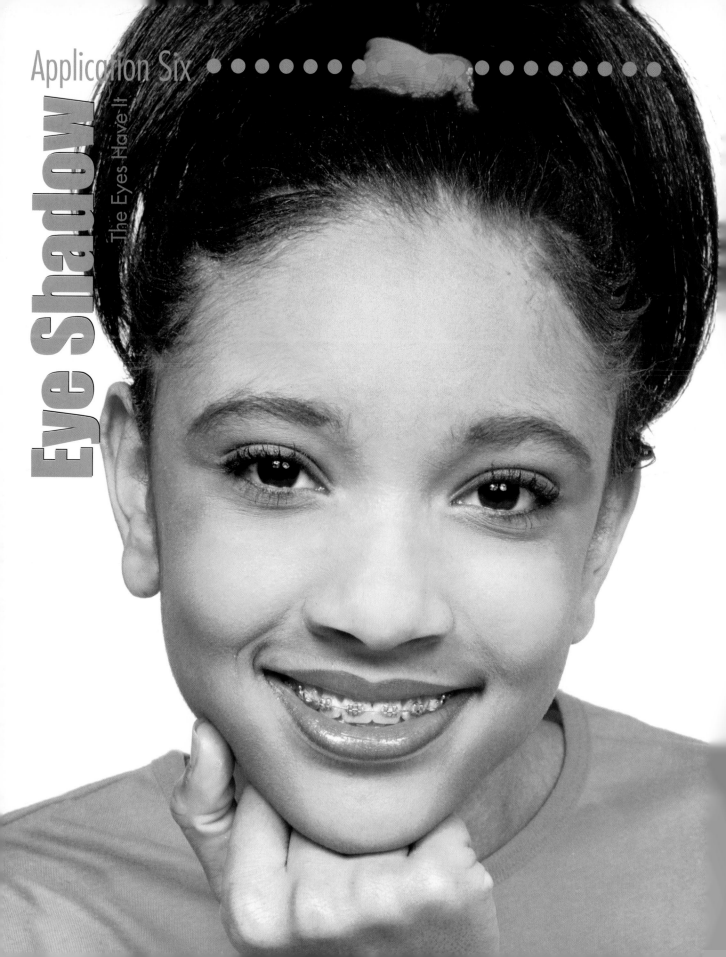

Eye Shadow

The Eyes Have It

Eye shadow is one of the most flexible and expressive cosmetics. It not only compliments your wardrobe, but it also portrays the mood you're trying to create for the day, night, or special occasion. Are you just waking up and going to school, or are you off to the prom? What does your eye shadow style convey? You can fashion a new and beautiful look simply by applying three basic shadows. There are a variety of application methods, each creating a different look. And with all the colors on the market, your possibilities are endless!

Eye shadow is an inexpensive way to have fun and be creative with color. You can try everything from natural hues to colorful shades of green, purple, and blue. Ready? Let's get started.

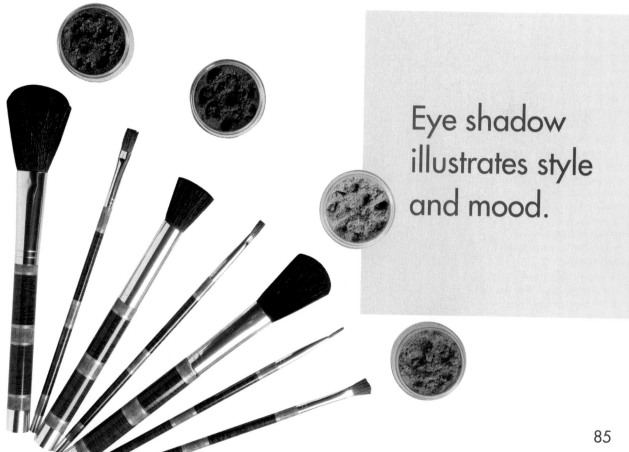

Eye shadow illustrates style and mood.

85

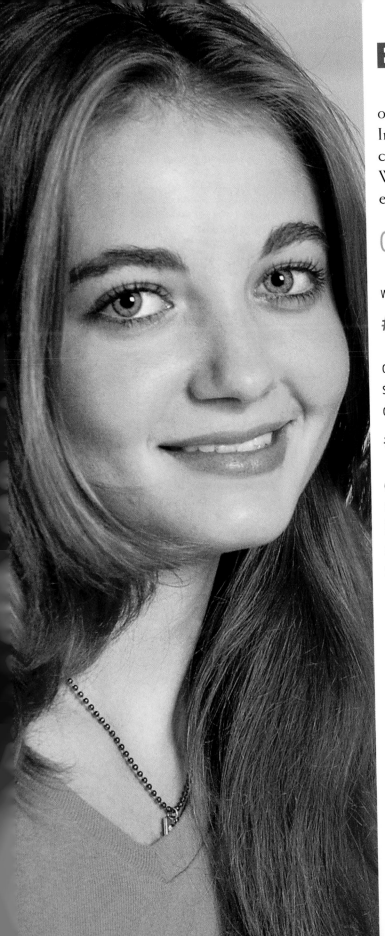

Eye Facts Unshadowed

There are countless *colors* of eye shadow on the market but a limited number of *kinds*. In this section we'll examine the pros and cons of each type of shadow available. We'll also learn how color can be used most effectively.

Check It Out

There are two things to consider when buying eye shadows: what kind to use and what colors you should apply.

#1: Kind

Eye shadow is packaged in powder, cream, liquid, wet/dry, or pencil form. I like powders the best because they go on smooth and are easy to blend. Make your choice based on the one that works well for you.

#2: Color

As you get started, you'll need three shadow colors that compliment one another and easily blend together: a light, medium, and dark shade. The lightest color you choose should be neutral since it will be used as a base color for your entire eye area. If you don't know where to begin, I suggest that you select earthy colors such as browns or grays.

Tammy's Tip
To enhance your eyes, find shadows that compliment your eye color; don't match your shadow to your iris.

The Answer Is

There are a variety of eye shadows packaged in many clever ways, everything from liquid wands to self-sharpening pencils. To eliminate some of the confusion, I've narrowed your selection to five basic kinds:

Powder: Powder shadows come in the widest color selection and are easy to apply and blend. The only aggravation I find with powder shadow is that it sometimes sprinkles beneath the eye. If this happens, use your makeup sponge and clean up the excess shadow dust when you're through.

Cream: Cream eye shadows are usually packaged in compacts or tubes, and are applied using your ring finger. They tend to be thick and pasty, creasing in the fold of your eye.

Liquid: Liquid eye shadow comes in wand form for easy application. It can also be purchased in a tube, which is best applied with your ring finger. It goes on smooth and creamy, but it also tends to crease in the fold of your eye.

Wet/Dry Shadows: Wet/dry shadows can be used either way, wet or dry. When used dry, they give a soft powder effect and when wet, the color becomes more intense. When wet shadow dries, it can be difficult to blend.

Pencils: Pencil eye shadows come in a variety of sizes. They can be large and chunky or smooth and sleek. Pencils allow you to draw the color on right where you want, but they can also tug on your eyelids. The oily emollients they're made of can easily cause smears, smudges, and creases.

Have fun and experiment with the different kinds of shadows, but keep two things in mind. You want them to blend and wear well without creasing.

Never feel embarrassed to tell the salesclerk if you don't like something they're trying to sell you. Honesty makes you a savvy shopper and saves money too.

Tammy's Tip • • • • • • • • • • • •
I found my best eye shadow colors in a free gift with purchase offer. In fact I've discovered many great cosmetic items that way.

Time Out with Tammy—

The first time I went to a department store for a makeover, I had quite an experience. I sat on the stool, anxiously awaiting the gal to complete her artistry. Finally she was finished. She proudly handed me a mirror as she raved about her work. I excitedly looked in the mirror . . . and gasped! My eyes made me look like Cat Woman!

She enthusiastically asked me what I thought. But I didn't know what to say without hurting her feelings. I muttered on, telling her what I liked until I finally mustered up the courage to tell her I didn't care for my eye makeup.

To my surprise, she wasn't put out at all. She happily changed it, and I went home a satisfied customer.

Beauty Bonus

If you don't know what colors to start with, I suggest purchasing an eye shadow kit that contains lots of colors to choose from. They are a relatively inexpensive way to experiment with colors you might never have dreamed of trying.

How It Applies

There are many ways to apply eye shadow. In this section I'm going to teach you how to apply the three same shadows—light, medium, and dark—in a number of different ways, each creating a different look.

Determine what kind of look you want. Below you'll find a variety of different ideas to try. Some of them improve the shape of the eyes, while others express your mood. The success of any application is to make sure you blend it well using an eye shadow brush. Unblended eye shadows look disconnected, breaking up the continuity of your eye.

All-Natural Gal Look—Apply the lightest shadow from the base of your lash line to your brow and then apply the medium shade in the crease of your lid. Gently blend.

Drama Queen Look—Apply the lightest shade from your lash line to your brow and then apply the darker shade over your lid. Blend upward from the crease.

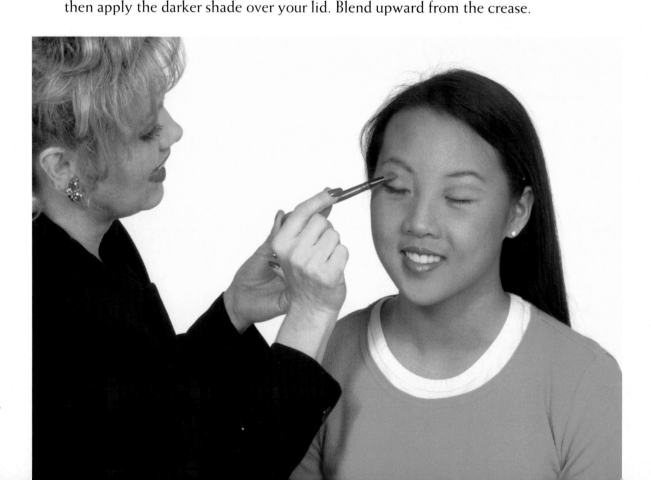

Flirty Chic Look—Apply the lightest shadow from your lashes to your brow and then apply the medium shadow to the inside corners of your eyelids and blend outward.

One Classy Lady Look—Apply the lightest color from your lash line to your brow and then apply the medium shade to the outer corner of your eyelids, blending upwards into the crease of your lid.

Close-set Eyes—Apply a neutral medium color from your lash line to your brow and then apply the darker shadow to the outer corners of your eyelids. Use the lightest shadow to accentuate the outer half of your brow bone and blend.

Wide-set Eyes—Apply a neutral medium shadow from your lash line to your brow and then apply the darkest shadow in the crease from the middle of your lid inward. Next, gently blend from the inside corner of your eye upwards to your brow. Highlight the outer two-thirds of your brow arch with the lightest shadow.

Deep-set Eyes—Apply a neutral medium shadow from your lash line to your brow and then apply the darker shadow just above the crease of your lid and blend upward. Apply the lightest shadow on your lid and just beneath your brow.

Small Narrow Eyes—Apply a neutral light shadow from your lash line to your brow. Then apply the medium shadow to your eyelid and the darkest shadow from the middle of your crease outward and blend.

Large Round Eyes—Apply a neutral medium shadow from your lash line to your brow. Apply the darkest shadow to the crease of your eye, blending outwards to the corner of your eye and then up. Highlight the base of your brow bone with the lightest shadow.

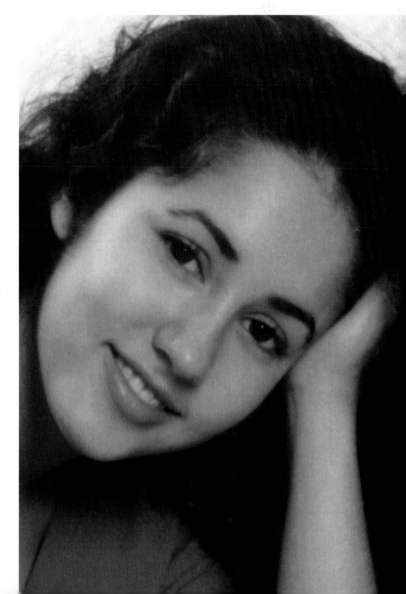

I once read a poll that asked guys and gals what they noticed about one another first, and the answer by both sexes was overwhelmingly the eyes. Now you have the insight you need to expertly improve your peepers, and your first impressions!

Putting It to the Test

Use the following form to measure the success of the shadows you sample. I suggest that you begin with three neutral shadows: light, medium, and dark. Try earth tones such as beiges, tans, grays, and peaches. Once you feel comfortable with applying eye shadow, experiment with different colors and have fun with it.

The key to unshadowing beautiful eyes is a good eye shadow.

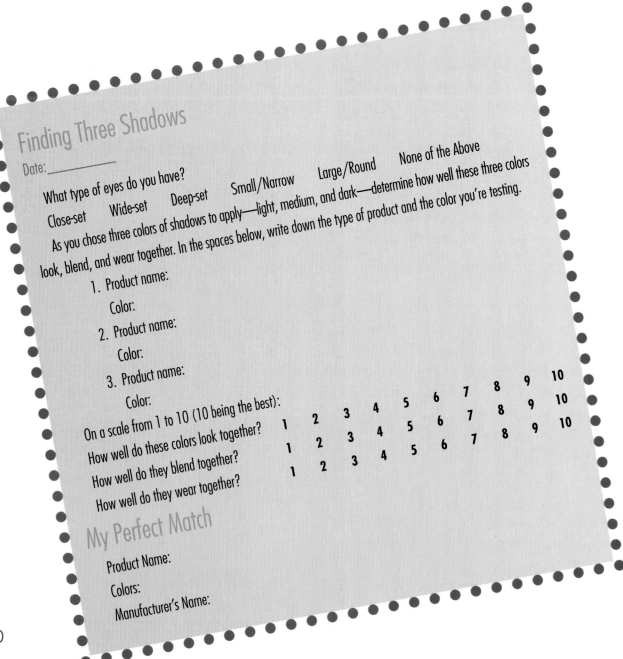

Finding Three Shadows

Date:_____

What type of eyes do you have?

Close-set   Wide-set   Deep-set   Small/Narrow   Large/Round   None of the Above

As you chose three colors of shadows to apply—light, medium, and dark—determine how well these three colors look, blend, and wear together. In the spaces below, write down the type of product and the color you're testing.

1. Product name:

   Color:

2. Product name:

   Color:

3. Product name:

   Color:

On a scale from 1 to 10 (10 being the best):

How well do these colors look together?   1   2   3   4   5   6   7   8   9   10

How well do they blend together?   1   2   3   4   5   6   7   8   9   10

How well do they wear together?   1   2   3   4   5   6   7   8   9   10

My Perfect Match

Product Name:

Colors:

Manufacturer's Name:

Eye shadow can be applied to accentuate the shape of your eyes or express a certain style. But the true expression of your eyes is found beneath the surface. All the makeup in the world can't hide the person you are on the inside. Your eyes openly convey your true feelings and emotions.

It's often said, "The eyes are the mirrors of our soul." Our eyes reveal so much about us. Just by looking at someone's eyes you can tell if they're sick, playful, hurting, happy, angry, or deep in thought. And if you're a Christian, your eyes should also reflect the love of God in your soul.

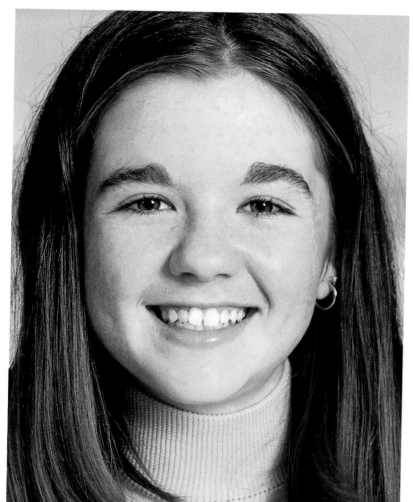

Shadow your eyes in the reflection of God's love.

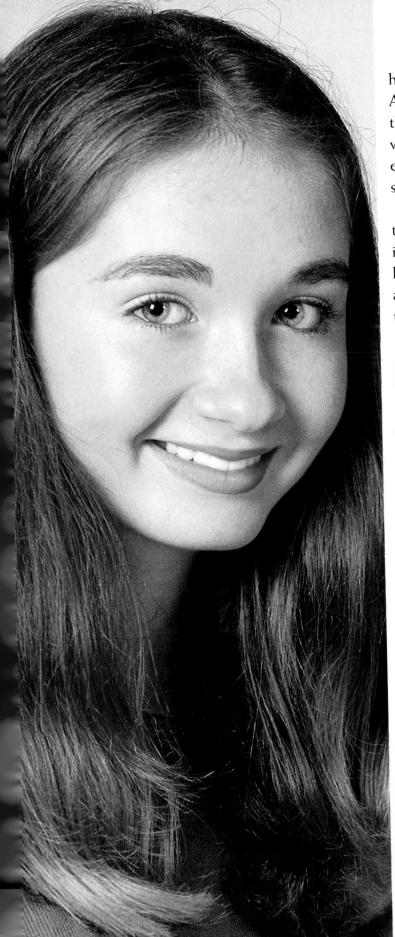

Reflecting God's love can be one of the hardest things Christians are called to do. After all, we're only human. We go through the same emotions as everyone else, and we're faced with the same temptations as everyone else. Yet we're called to a higher standard of living than anyone else. Is it fair?

In this part of the application, we're going to focus on how our eyes play such an important role in our Christian lives. We'll learn how to accentuate the positive and alleviate the negative by shadowing some of the things we see.

Eye Facts Unshadowed

Have you ever heard the children's song, *O Be Careful Little Eyes What You See?*
The words of the song go like this:

O be careful little eyes what you see,
O be careful little eyes what you see,
For the Father up above is looking down
*   with love,*
So be careful little eyes what you see.

Though you may have sung it as a child, the words still apply as you grow older, especially during your teenage years. Satan tempts us visually today more than ever before. We have become a highly visual generation through movies, video games, music videos, magazines, television, and the computer. We tend to think that we're mindless when participating in these activities, but that isn't true. Our consciences slowly become seared when we watch, look at, and see things we shouldn't. We start adapting to the world's way of thinking. And we move away from biblical morals or adapt them to accommodate our culture.

Did you know that years ago, during the time of war, men were made to watch violent, gruesome movies (like today's television) to prepare them for combat? The government's goal was to make them so unfeeling to blood, death, and life that they would forget reality and carry out their mission without their conscience telling them to do otherwise. This method of desensitization still works. After the school shooting at Columbine, I saw an interview with a student who had witnessed the violence. He commented, "It didn't seem real. I felt like I was watching TV."

I know the same thing has happened to me. I once drove past a deadly accident where bloody bodies laid draped in cloth at the side of the road while rescue workers used the jaws of life to free someone from the twisted wreckage. I looked on with little feeling, not realizing what actually happened. I had seen it on TV so many times that I was numb to the real tragedy and devastation that was right before me.

Or what about 9-11? The images of those jets crashing into the World Trade Towers didn't seem real. It was like watching another *Die Hard* movie. It literally took me a couple of days to comprehend the devestating reality of what took place because Hollywood has had a numbing effect on my mind.

We're visually programmed by the media to accept the unacceptable and justify the unjustifiable. We lose all sense of reality and become blinded to good and bad by our very own eyes.

Check It Out

Our eyes not only desensitize us to sin, they also lure us into it. As the saying goes, "Garbage in, garbage out." What we take in through our eyes starts affecting the way we think. And once it affects our thought process, it will affect the way we act.

In recent years, Hollywood has started dealing with the supernatural, demons, witchcraft, and astrology. Many teens are investigating the mystique of the dark side after seeing it favorably portrayed by TV and movies. Christian teens have been affected as well.

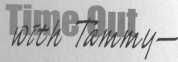
Time-Out
with Tammy—

I used to watch soap operas all the time. I didn't miss an episode if I could help it, and if I couldn't fit them into my schedule, I videotaped them. I was addicted.

I remember the very first soap I watched. It involved a married man and woman who were having an affair with one another. The hot and steamy scene piqued my interest so much that I couldn't wait for the next episode to air. Over and over again I watched sex, rape, murder, robbery, and many other scandalous affairs. Soon I became so absorbed that it all seemed perfectly acceptable.

After we repeatedly see something over and over again we become immune to it. At first we might be shocked or sickened, but after awhile we don't have those feelings anymore. We eventually become indifferent to right and wrong.

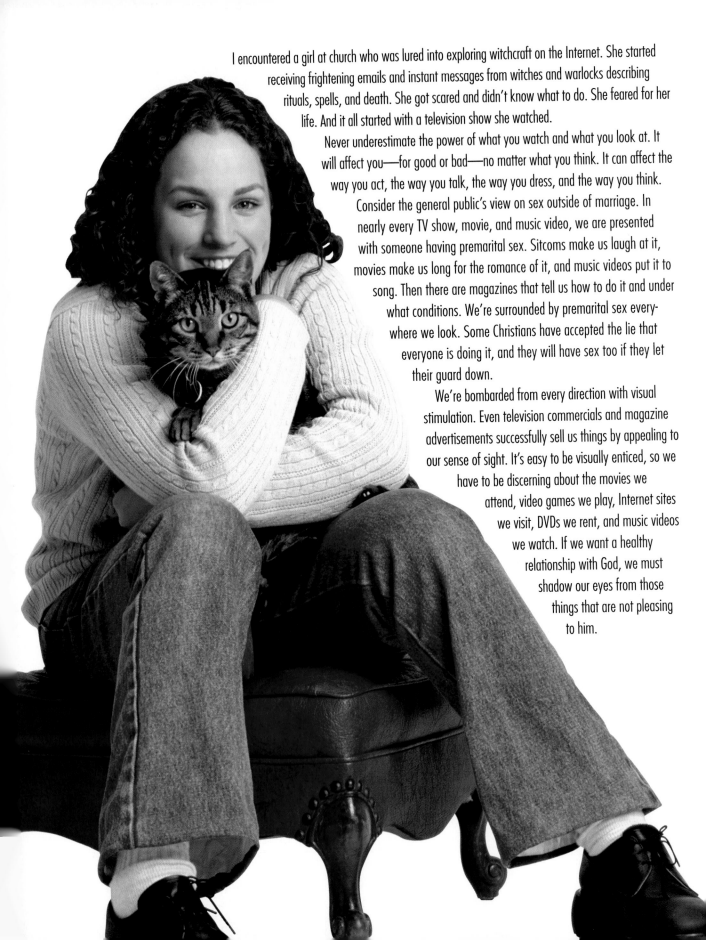

I encountered a girl at church who was lured into exploring witchcraft on the Internet. She started receiving frightening emails and instant messages from witches and warlocks describing rituals, spells, and death. She got scared and didn't know what to do. She feared for her life. And it all started with a television show she watched.

Never underestimate the power of what you watch and what you look at. It will affect you—for good or bad—no matter what you think. It can affect the way you act, the way you talk, the way you dress, and the way you think. Consider the general public's view on sex outside of marriage. In nearly every TV show, movie, and music video, we are presented with someone having premarital sex. Sitcoms make us laugh at it, movies make us long for the romance of it, and music videos put it to song. Then there are magazines that tell us how to do it and under what conditions. We're surrounded by premarital sex everywhere we look. Some Christians have accepted the lie that everyone is doing it, and they will have sex too if they let their guard down.

We're bombarded from every direction with visual stimulation. Even television commercials and magazine advertisements successfully sell us things by appealing to our sense of sight. It's easy to be visually enticed, so we have to be discerning about the movies we attend, video games we play, Internet sites we visit, DVDs we rent, and music videos we watch. If we want a healthy relationship with God, we must shadow our eyes from those things that are not pleasing to him.

The Answer Is

Matthew 6:22–23—The eye is the lamp of the body. If your eyes are good, your whole body will be full of light. But if your eyes are bad, your whole body will be full of darkness. If then the light within you is darkness, how great is that darkness!

Your eyes are a window to your body. Not only do you see out, but others also see in. In Matthew 6, Jesus says, "If therefore your eyes are good, your whole body will be full of light. But if your eyes are bad, your whole body will be full of darkness." One way or another, our eyes have a lot to say about us.

Remember reading Matthew 5:14 and 16 in application 4? There Jesus said, "You are the light of the world . . . let your light so shine before men, that they may see your good deeds and praise your Father in heaven." This verse is connected with the one in Matthew 6. When your eyes are good and filled with the light of God's love, you are a bright light to the world. But when you're not living the way God wants you to, your light is flickering in darkness.

You can tell a lot about a person by their eyes. When the eyes are good, the whole body is good, and when the eyes are bad, the whole body is bad. If someone's eyes are angry their whole body is angry, and if their eyes are sad their whole body is sad. Understand? Even people who don't know you can look into your eyes and see what lies beneath the surface. But it's difficult for them to see the light of God's love and acceptance when you're out of his will.

I've been dressed up with perfect makeup, hair, and nails, thinking no one would notice that I was hurting inside. But total strangers would approach me and ask if I was okay. They said, "Your eyes look so sad." Underneath all that makeup I wasn't hiding a thing.

Our parents, close friends, and relatives have a knack for knowing what's going on by looking into our eyes. I can't count the times my mother looked into my eyes and said, "Tammy Sue, you're lying." My eyes didn't fool her, no matter how clever I thought I was.

The last sentence of Matthew 6:23 says, "If then the light within you is darkness, how great is that darkness!" What does this mean to you? I think it means we can get lost in our own sin. We watch the lies that are filtered through the media— everyone is having sex, homosexuality is natural, abortion is a choice—and we start to believe them without a second thought. That's the way sin operates. At first we know we're wrong, but after we do it for awhile we become immune to it. We get lost in our own darkness, and great is the darkness! When we're lost in the dark and can't find our way, how can we possibly lead others in the right direction?

Time Out with Tammy—

I skipped school my junior year of high school and lied to cover it up. I thought, "That was easy. I'm off the hook." That lie worked so well, I started lying about other things. And pretty soon I was lying to cover up my lies! I forgot where the truth started and the lying began. In fact, I justified it so well I started believing my own lies! I became blinded to what I was doing and was lost in the darkness of lying.

Luckily, I got caught. I suffered some major humiliation, but in the long run I got right with God. However, that wasn't the end of it. My parents and teachers now looked into my eyes wondering if they could trust me. They looked for the light of honesty to shine from within.

Tammy's Tip •••••••••• Shelter your eyes from sin to protect your light within.

95

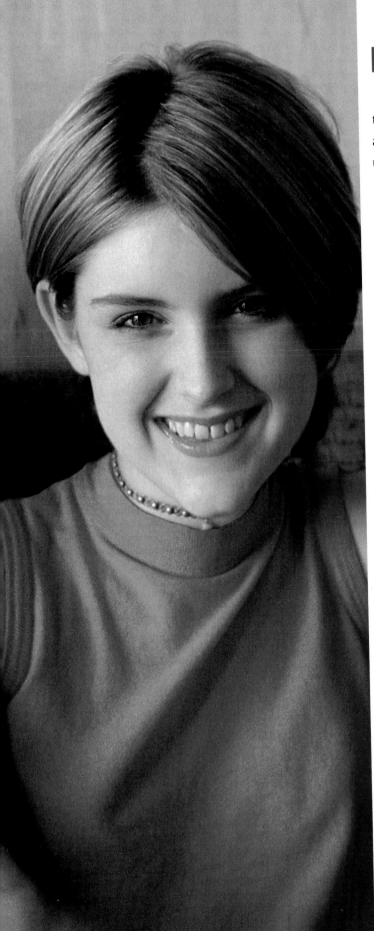

Beauty Bonus

There are many verses in the Bible that talk about light. Many of them refer to Jesus as "the light" (John 1). While others refer to us as "children of light" (Ephesians 5).

When you accept Jesus as your Lord and Savior, the Holy Spirit shines within you making you a child of light.

God is our power source. Our lights glow brightly when we're close to him, but tend to weaken when we move toward sin. When you talk on a cordless phone, you can hear well as long as you stay close to the base. But when you get outside the base's range, the voice on the other end starts breaking up and it's hard to hear. God is our base. As long as we stay within his range, our light shines bright, but when we move too far away, our light dims and it's hard to see. As soon as we move back toward God, our signal glows strong again.

How It Applies

Remember when I said, "Reflecting God's love can be one of the hardest things Christians are called to do"? It's true. We may be Christians, but we're tempted by sin like everyone else. The same eyes that are supposed to show God's love and acceptance lure us into sin. So what can we do?

I've found prayer highly effective in this area of my life. I ask God to help me avoid the temptation to sin. And I ask him to make me loving and accepting through his love and acceptance.

By nature I am not a loving, accepting, and compassionate person. My family and friends will tell you that I have to work hard at it. I pray almost daily, "Lord let my eyes show your love and compassion for others." Even as a teen I prayed that I would accept others for who they were, not who I wanted them to be. As a result my heart changed toward Roy, a mentally handicapped boy at school. I had hated that he sat behind me and always wanted to talk to me. He drooled all the time and often wiped his nose with his deformed hand and then patted me on the back. If that wasn't bad enough, I got paired up with Roy as my square dance partner in PE. That's when I prayed and asked God to forgive me for disliking Roy and to give me a new square dance partner. Instead, God changed my heart towards Roy. I learned that he wasn't so bad after all. Underneath that unapproachable exterior was one terrific human being. God didn't give me a new partner; he gave Roy a new partner by changing my attitude.

Putting It to the Test

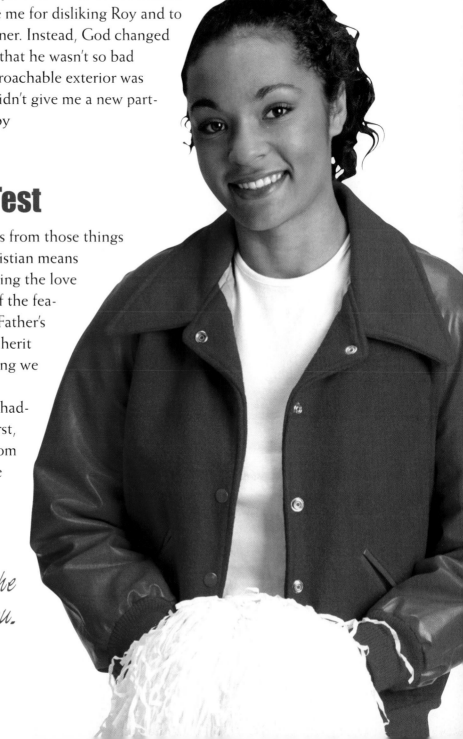

It's up to us to shadow our eyes from those things that tempt us to sin. Being a Christian means becoming Christ-like and mirroring the love of God through our eyes. One of the features I pray you acquire is your "Father's eyes." Unfortunately, we don't inherit them naturally—they're something we have to seek after.

Remember there are two eye shadows we can ask God to apply. First, "Lord, please shadow my eyes from temptation." And second, "Please shadow them in your love and acceptance of others."

Beauty Secret #6:
Eye shadow expresses the
"Super Model" in you.

Eyelashes

Extending Your Potential

I can't count the times I've heard it said, "Just bat your pretty eyelashes," suggesting that this will get you whatever you want. Maybe that's the reason so many of us desire those long, lush beauties. Very few are blessed with thick, intense eyelashes, but fortunately there are many products on the market to help our lashes reach their fullest potential. In this application we're going to take a look at how you can lengthen short lashes, thicken fine lashes, and define and separate each one for precise individuality. With a little know-how you'll have those babies fluttering in no time!

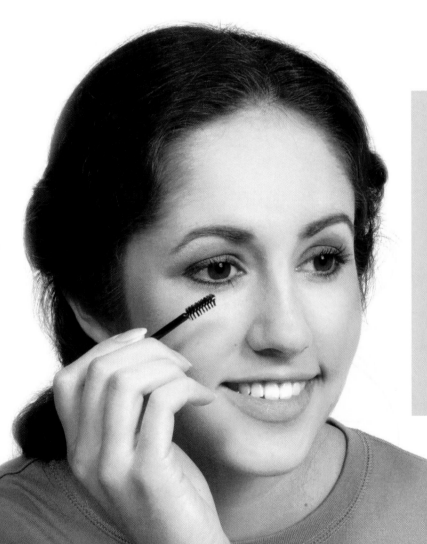

Long, lush lashes illuminate your eyes.

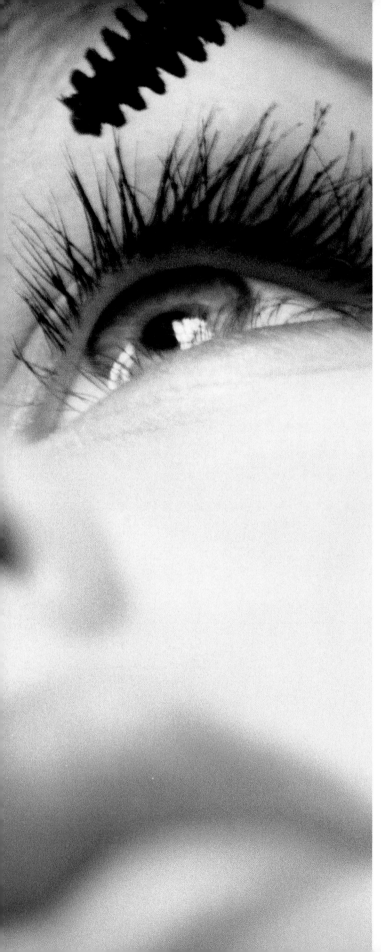

There are many items on the market that make optimistic but outrageous claims. I know because I've tried them all. After seeing a television commercial, I once ran to the store and bought mascara that would allegedly curl my lashes without a curler. And then there was the magazine advertisement that sold me on vitamin-enriched gel that would make my lashes grow longer overnight. I hate to admit it, but I've fallen for gimmick after gimmick, hoping that I would end up with fully defined, feathery soft, smudge resistant, luscious lashes that set in seconds. After years of purchasing useless products, I've grown poorer but wiser. Read on and learn for yourself how to spot false claims and understand the fine points of a product.

Facts for Fuller Lashes

There are a variety of mascaras on the market with different additives and applicators designed to lengthen, thicken, and condition. And if you like to play with color, you can buy mascara in funky colors too! Let's take a look at what the makeup industry has to offer.

Check It Out

Cosmetics manufacturers are bustling with different lash-making legends. It's up to you to create your own happily-ever-after story by finding the mascara that works best for your lashes. To get started you'll need to answer two basic questions: What kind do you need? and What color do you want?

#1: Kind

What do you want your mascara to do for you? Do you want it to lengthen, thicken, or condition your lashes? The ingredients

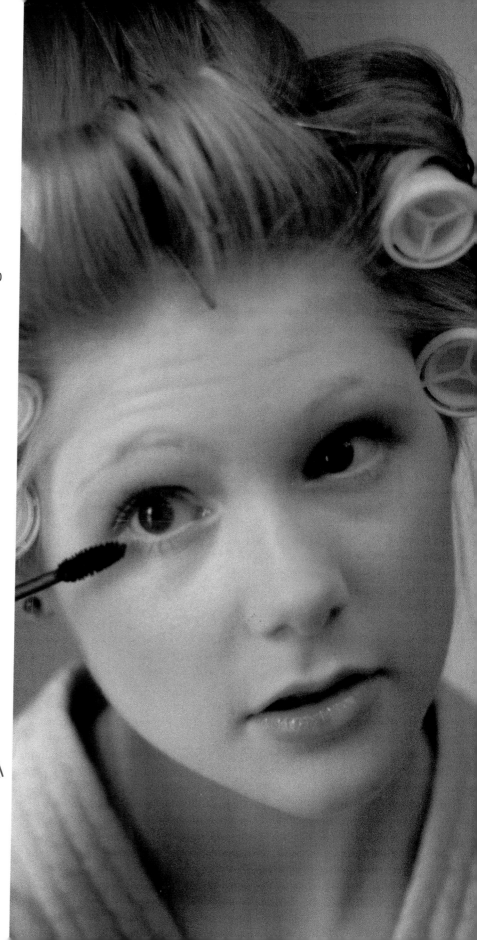

for lengthening and thickening are similar, but the applicators are usually different. For example, if you have long lashes, you'll need mascara with a full brush that separates and thickens each lash. Keep in mind that the applicator is very important to the overall effectiveness of the mascara.

#2: Color

Mascara comes in a broad range of colors, everything from ravenous black to peacock blue. I would recommend that you pick a basic color such as brown or brown/black for everyday wear and choose brighter colors such as purples and greens for those special occasions.

The Answer Is

There are six types of mascara to choose from, and their success or failure is generally determined by the applicator. To help you understand how applicators work, I have included applicator information along with descriptions of various mascara formulas.

Tammy's Tip • • • •
Most teens look best in brown or brown/black mascara. (If your hair color is black, then black mascara will be your natural choice.)

My girlfriend, Dana, plucked her eyelashes out because someone told her they would grow back longer and thicker. Much to her distress, they didn't grow back at all. Dana learned to expertly apply false eyelashes, and if you met her today, you would never know that she was lashless. Her secret? She trims the lashes before she glues them on, making them look imperfect and natural. She then applies two coats of mascara and is able to make one set of false eyelashes last for three to four weeks.

Tammy's Tip
If you have light-colored lashes such as blonde or red, apply mascara to the top side of your upper lashes first, and then apply it to their underside. This gives your lashes complete rich color.

Lengthening: Lengthening mascara is designed to make short lashes appear longer.

Thickening: Thickening mascara will give your lashes volume. It's a bit heavier than lengthening mascara and may form clumps.

Conditioning: Conditioning mascaras can be found in lengthening and thickening forms. They contain vitamin complexes that promote soft, plump, healthy eyelashes.

Waterproof: Waterproof mascara stays on when you swim, sweat, and sob. It is heavier and thicker than regular mascara, so it may dry and break your lashes with prolonged use. To remove waterproof mascara, use eye-safe makeup remover.

Color: Colored mascaras come in an array of trendy colors. They can be found in regular and waterproof formulas.

Clear: Clear mascara is a conditioning gel that glosses and thickens lashes without adding color. You can use clear mascara on your eyelashes as well as your eyebrows.

Hypoallergenic: Hypoallergenic mascara is formulated for sensitive eyes and for those who wear contacts.

Full Bristle Brush: This is my favorite brush. Its thick bristles lengthen, separate, and feather eyelashes without clumping.

Multitiered Brush: This brush is designed to build and separate lashes. If you're not careful, it may clump lashes with two or more coats of mascara.

Twisted Brush: This brush is difficult to use. You need to gently roll it up your lashes as you apply the mascara to receive a full application and avoid clumping.

Curved Brush: This brush is intended to curl your lashes as you apply your mascara, but it doesn't seem to work well. It's also difficult to use on tiny lashes in the corner of your eyes.

Eyelash Comb: Eyelash combs separate and define long lashes but tend to clump thick lashes. They work best when used before mascara dries, because they can get caught in dry lashes and pull them out.

Beauty Bonus

When your eyelashes just don't seem to cut it, you may want to try false eyelashes. There are two types: single lashes and a full strip of lashes. The single lashes are used to fill in individual spots where your own lashes are lacking, while full strip lashes are applied across the entire length of the upper eyelid. False eyelashes of any kind can be difficult to apply, but after some practice you'll figure out how to put them on and take them off with minimal time and effort. I recommend that you buy a kit, follow the manufacturer's directions, and practice, practice, practice until you're comfortable with how they look and feel.

How It Applies

Applying mascara is pretty easy, but there are some techniques you can use to help your lashes reach their fullest potential. The steps below will have your lashes looking full and fabulous in no time!

Curl Lashes—The first step to beautiful lashes is curling them with an eyelash curler. Curl them before you apply mascara to avoid lash breakage. With the curler opened, place your upper lashes in the opening, positioning the curler at the root. With a steady hand, gently squeeze the curler shut, hold ten seconds, and release.

Twist, Don't Pump—Without removing the wand, unscrew the mascara and slowly twist the brush around to coat the bristles. Don't pump the wand up and down, this allows air into the tube and dries out the mascara.

Tammy's Tip • • • • • • • • • •
To intensify the look of colored mascara, layer it over your regular color.

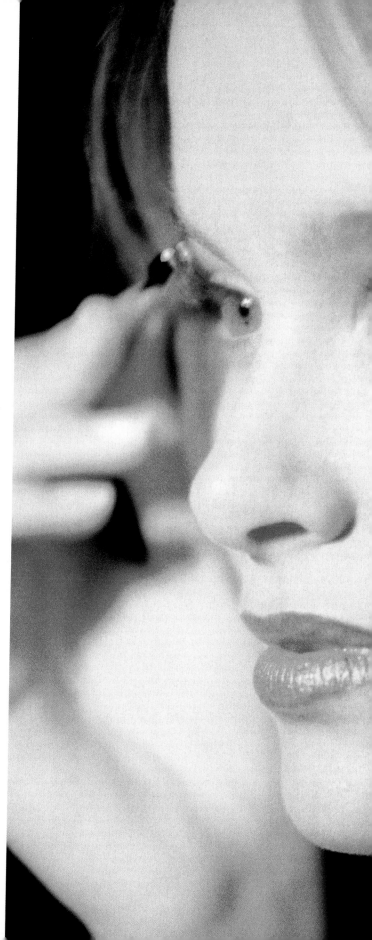

Apply Mascara—Position the brush at the base of your upper lashes and gently sweep upward to the tip of your lashes. Repeat this process on your lower lashes. To avoid clumping, apply a second coat of mascara before the first coat dries.

Flakes and Clumps—To remove flakes and clumps, use a clean mascara brush. I kept a wand from an empty mascara tube, which I washed and use just for this purpose.

Smudges—To clean up smudges, use the narrow end of a makeup wedge or a Q-tip. A light application of translucent powder under your eye prevents mascara from rubbing off or smudging.

Putting It to the Test

Use the following form to determine the success of each mascara you try. Also note the kind of brush each brand provides, whether or not it was easy to use, and if the mascara applied without clumping.

The key to unleashing great-looking lashes is found in mascara.

Finding My Mascara

Date: _____

1. Product name:
   Color:
   Type of Brush:
   Looks Good: **YES / NO**
   Clumps: **YES / NO**
   Easy to Apply: **YES / NO**

2. Product name:
   Color:
   Type of Brush:
   Looks Good: **YES / NO**
   Clumps: **YES / NO**
   Easy to Apply: **YES / NO**

Product name:
   Color:
   Type of Brush:
   Looks Good: **YES / NO**
   Clumps: **YES / NO**
   Easy to Apply: **YES / NO**

My Perfect Match

Product Name:
Type of Brush:
Manufacturer's Name:

We use everything from colored mascara to rich vitamin E oil on our eyelashes to enhance them. We resort to false eyelashes when our own just won't do. And we even meticulously separate each and every lash to give individuality and fullness to the overall effect of our eyelashes.

In part two of this application we're going to look at how you can define and accentuate your talents. Just as you've learned to enhance your eyelashes to compliment your eyes, you can develop and enhance your individual talents to bring glory to God.

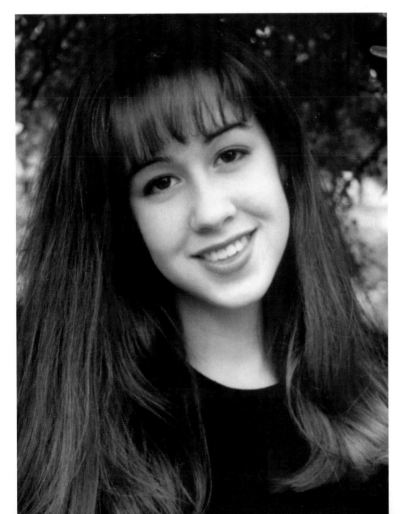

Extend your talents in a way that illuminates praise for God.

105

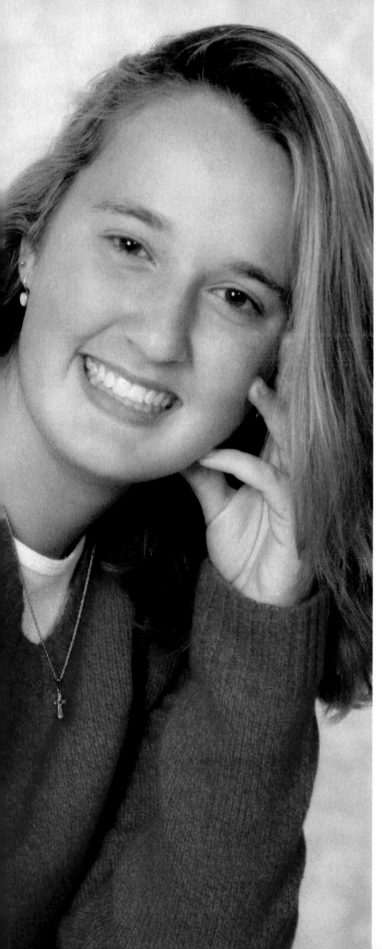

We spend valuable time and money on beauty magazines, researching beauty secrets of super models and stars. But I'm afraid we spend less time developing and caring for one another with the individual gifts God has given us. Our physical beauty passes with time, but the internal beauty that we share through our talents can last a lifetime. Whether it's singing a song to touch someone's heart or volunteering to baby-sit for a tired mom, we each have individual abilities that can touch a life and bring praise to God.

Facts for Fuller Life

God has given us our own unique gifts and talents. Yes, that includes you too! Many of us fail to recognize our own abilities and therefore fail to use them. We tend to think, "If I could only play the piano like Liberace or sing like Madonna, then I would have something to pass on. But I can't so I guess I'll do nothing."

Gifts and talents come in many packages. Some are wrapped up in a song and others are a present of encouraging words. Maybe your special gifts come in the form of raking leaves for a shut-in, baking cookies for a new neighbor, tutoring someone in math, or sending a card to brighten a friend's day. Each of us has our own unique talent. Use the abilities you already have, rather than downplaying your talent and wishing you were someone else.

If you don't know what your special abilities are, use the following questionnaire to define your skills.

Check It Out

What do you enjoy doing in your spare time?
What are your hobbies?
What is your favorite subject in school?
Do you play a musical instrument?
What extracurricular activities do you participate in?
What are your interests?
What are your career goals?
What do your friends say your talents are?
What do your parents say your talents are?
Is there an area of service you enjoy or have wanted to try?
How could you put your gifts and interests to work?

The Answer Is

Once you discover your gifts, you'll find blessing in giving them away.

1 Peter 4:10 (NKJV)—As each one has received a gift, minister it to one another, as good stewards of the manifold grace of God.

Read 1 Peter 4:10 one more time in the New International Version:

1 Peter 4:10—Each one should use whatever gift he has received to serve others, faithfully administrating God's grace in its various forms.

It's not about what your abilities *are* as much as it's about how you *use* them. All of us have different talents that we can share with others, but it's up to us to use what we've been given. The true success of our talent is found on the inside of who we are. What do I mean by that? You must be willing to openheartedly share of yourself.

I've known individuals with marvelous talents that they never shared with anybody. They never willingly gave of themselves without being paid. Payment isn't always a bad thing, but when it's the only thing that motivates you to give of yourself, you might want to reexamine who you are beneath the surface. I've known girls who won't lift a finger at home without the promise of cash, new clothes, or something else they want. That's selfish greed, not selfless giving.

When was the last time you did something just because? You could help your mom with the housework without being asked. Or you could do the dishes for your brother or

Time Out with Tammy—

As you review your list, keep in mind you may have talents that you never thought of. I have always been interested in makeup, poise, and etiquette. And nearly every report card I received stated, "Tammy tends to talk too much." I overlooked these abilities for years, not realizing they were actually gifts I could use to serve others. God turned my talents into MakeOver Ministries, and he can use your talents too. Don't be tempted to think what you do is insignificant. God can use anything you're willing to give, and then he gives back to you! Every time I use my talents to touch a life, the blessings come back to me. It's like putting a dollar into your savings account and going back the next day to find your one dollar turned into ten. What a great feeling!

Go back to Check It Out and look at your list again to see if there's anything you've overlooked.

Tammy's Tip . . . .
What do capability, availability, accountability, and responsibility all have in common? Ability, ability, ability, ability!

sister even though it isn't your turn. You could even mow the yard for Dad without being prompted. Now maybe you're thinking, "What kind of talents are those?" But remember what I said earlier: It's not about what your abilities *are* as much as it's about how you *use* them. Ability starts with capability and availability, which leads to responsibility. We must be responsible with what we've been given, including our time and talents.

Beauty Bonus

Now that you know you're capable, accountable, and responsible for making yourself available, how are you going to use your abilities? There are so many things you can do; it's just a matter of deciding where to start. Remember, you shouldn't be serving just to get special recognition for what you do. But your service can be noted on college and employment applications. Colleges love to see voluntary community service projects listed on your application, and even cleaning a little country church is a community service project!

Let's look at some creative ways you could put your gifts and talents to work.

Choir—Do you like to sing? It doesn't matter if you're an expert or not—the church choir is usually looking for willing voices, not necessarily professional ones.

Homeless Shelter—Homeless shelters are always looking for volunteers to serve food, collect and separate donations, and many other routine tasks.

Sandbagging—I grew up near a river that would swell outside its banks at least once a year. The local volunteer fire department was always looking for volunteers to fill sandbags. My friends and I had a great time helping out and playing in the sand!

Political Campaigns—Are you interested in politics? Volunteering at a local campaign headquarters is a great way to meet people and learn about politics on local, state, and national levels.

Time Out
with Tammy—

I was privileged to have parents that taught me about giving at an early age. I didn't like it at the time, but years later I came to appreciate what I was taught.

I grew up in a small town with a little country church. Our little church required janitorial services, someone to clean the church. Now, unlike the majority of churches today, this was not a paid position but a voluntary position filled by those within the church. My family, along with other church members, dedicated one Saturday every six weeks to polishing the pews, emptying the trash, cleaning the bathrooms, washing the bedding and toys in the nursery, sweeping the porch, mowing the lawn, weeding, and anything else that needed to be done. It was literally an all-day process. At the time I hated giving up my Saturdays, which I usually spent at the roller rink, to clean the church. How boring was that!

But I learned a great deal from the Saturdays I invested my time in. You'll think I'm nuts, but I actually look back upon them fondly.

Nursery—The church nursery is always looking for volunteers and so are tired mothers. I suggest taking a baby-sitting certification class from your local Red Cross chapter.

Car Wash—Organize your friends for a fun-filled water day. Car washes are usually fundraisers, but they don't have to be. They can be a great service project. Create a list of people that might not be capable of washing their own cars and start a traveling car wash.

Dog Wash—Wash your own dog or someone else's. Just be sure to muzzle them so they don't bite!

Blood Bank—If you're old enough, donate blood. You're not just giving blood— you're giving life.

Trash Pickup—Organize a group to pick up trash on the highway. Your local chamber of commerce can put you in touch with bags and reflector vests so you are safe.

Rake and Run—Plan a Saturday in the fall to rake leaves with your friends. Get a list of people that could use your help and make a day of it. Rake one yard and then run to the next. Top off the day with hot apple cider and cookies.

Nursing Home—I've always found the nursing home a rewarding way to serve others. On Sunday afternoons, my friend Jim would play his guitar, and we would join him in song. We weren't a hot group, but our audience sure loved us!

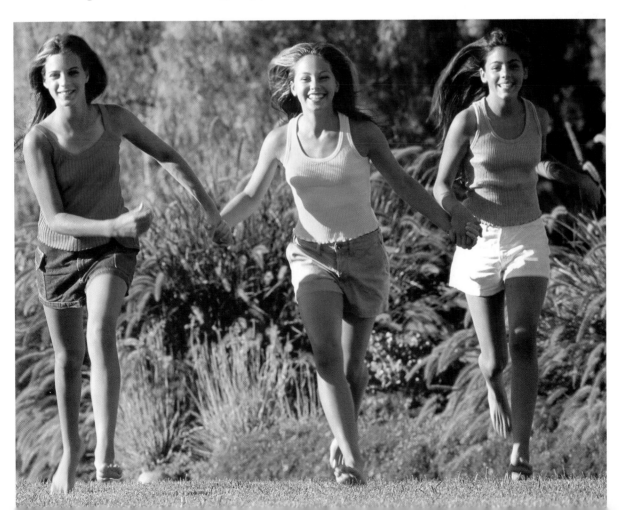

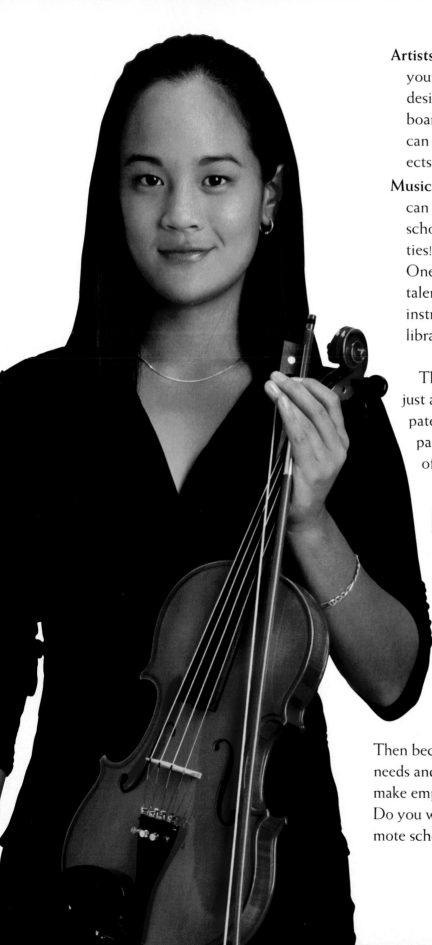

Artists—There are always ways to put your artwork to use. I've been able to design the church bulletin, bulletin boards, and business stationary. You can also organize children's craft projects for clubs, churches, and camps.

Musicians—There are many places you can volunteer your talent. Church, school, nursing homes, and even parties! My son is an awesome musician. One of the things he's done with his talent has involved introducing musical instruments to children at the local library fair.

The list goes on and on. These are just a few ideas that I've actually participated in. Ask your parents, teachers, pastor, counselor, or local chamber of commerce for more ideas.

How It Applies

Like our eyelashes, we must extend our talents in order to reach our greatest potential. As Christians we are to be Christlike, and Christ came to serve, not to be served. In fact, the key to successful leadership is being a servant first.

Do you want to be class president? Then become aware of what your class needs and find a way to take care of it; don't make empty promises just to get elected. Do you want to be a cheerleader? Then promote school pride by cleaning up the campus or encouraging others off the field. Do you want to be first chair clarinet? Then practice, study hard, and help others with their instruments. Do you want to be a star athlete? Then train, work positively with other teammates, and thank your coach for his or her dedication. Humbly put yourself in a place of service in order to become a true leader.

Matthew 23:11—"The greatest among you will be your servant."

Putting It to the Test

Define your talent, develop it, and extend it to its fullest potential. There are numerous ways you can share your gifts with others. Just as your eyelashes serve the purpose of protecting your eyes from tiny particles, your talents and abilites are given to serve a purpose as well.

When you give the gift of yourself, you also give yourself a gift in return. There is nothing more awe inspiring than applause and appreciation for sharing a part of your heart with others. And remember, even when your efforts go unnoticed here on earth, God notices everything.

Use your talents to reach out and attend to the needs of others and bring glory to God. Remember your cap*ability* and avail*ability* gives you account*ability* and respons*ibility* for your own ability.

Beauty Secret #7: Your lashes and talents define and extend the "Super Model" in you.

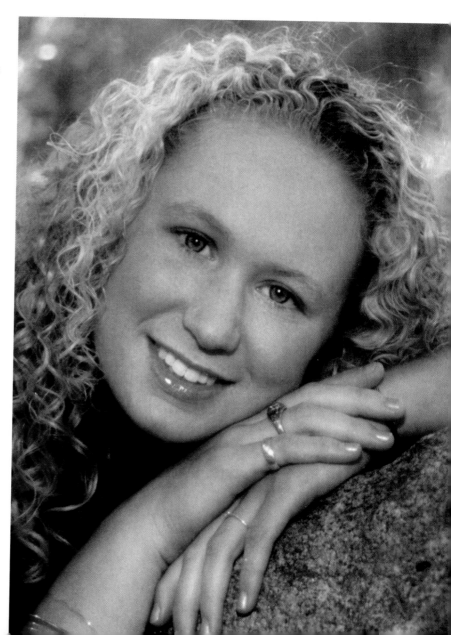

Eyebrows

Brow-Raising Results

Well-maintained eyebrows are the crowning touch to your eyes. Beautifully groomed brows give stylish shape, balance, detail, and drama to your face.

I'm often asked, "Should I pluck my brows or leave them alone? I'm afraid of getting them uneven." In this application, I'm going to take the guesswork out of eyebrow maintenance. We'll learn up-to-date techniques that will shape, style, and sketch beautiful brows into existence.

We often spend a great deal of time putting on our makeup each day, yet we tend to skip over an important part of the process—those pesky eyebrows. We don't know what to do with them, so we do nothing at all. Tweezing them is painful, waxing them is costly, and trimming them evenly seems better left to the pros. Sound confusing? Don't despair. Grab a cold drink from the fridge and read on!

Beautiful brows have a crowning effect.

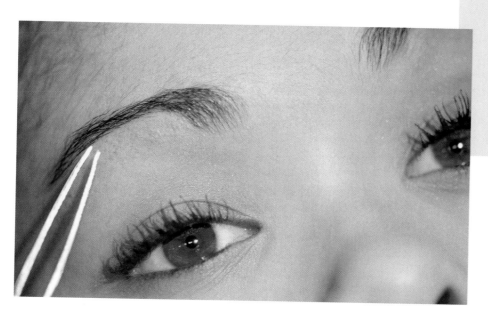

Brow-Raising Facts

Like other makeup products, companies offer different solutions for eyebrow care. You can purchase pencils and stencils to make application easier. And if that's not enough, there's professional waxing, bleaching, and dying. You have plenty of options; you just need to know where to begin.

Before we talk about products, we need to define the shape of your brows. Shaping your brows will enlarge small eyes, open up close-set and deep-set eyes, pull together wide-set eyes, and shape round eyes. So before we get started refer to application 5 to determine the shape of your eyes.

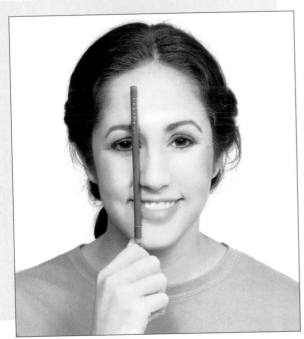

Before you apply any product, you need to shape up. You can either have your brows shaped professionally or you can follow the directions below and style them yourself.

For starters, it's best to tweeze eyebrows after you've showered. Hot water opens your pores, allowing the hair to be removed more easily. Use a quality pair of tweezers, pull your skin taut, and pluck individual hairs at the base with sharp swift movement in the direction they grow.

To determine where your brows should begin and end, look in a mirror and hold a pencil vertically against your nostril, aligning it with the inner corner of your eye (see photo above). This is where your brow should begin. Next leave the pencil against your nostril but move it at an angle to the outer corner of your eye (see photo at right). This will show you where your brow should end.

Start with those unruly hairs that grow blatantly outside the brow line. Next begin

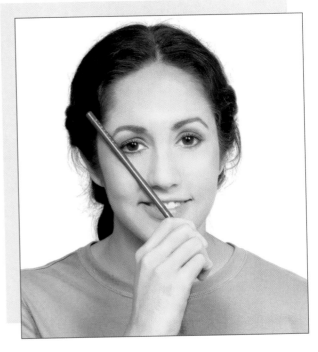

at the inner corner and work outward plucking hairs one by one as you carefully scrutinize your work after each one. Be careful not to pluck hairs above the brow line because it spoils the natural arch of the brow. Tweezing your brows doesn't remove the hair permanently, so your brows will need constant maintenance. However, sometimes tweezing your brows will prevent the hair follicles from reproducing.

Close-set Eyes—Remove just a few hairs from the inner part of the brow to create a sense of width.

Wide-set Eyes—Do not tweeze inner brows near your nose. Tweeze only the outer end of brows.

Deep-set Eyes—Remove hairs one by one on the underside of the brow, thinning out the thicker areas.

Small Narrow Eyes—Thin out heavy brows to open up small eyes.

Large Round Eyes—Do not thin brows. Only remove hairs growing outside the natural brow line.

Tammy's Tip • • • • • • • • • • • • • •
It's very important to tweeze only one hair at a time. Stand back and check your look before you tweeze others. You don't want to overtweeze your brows.

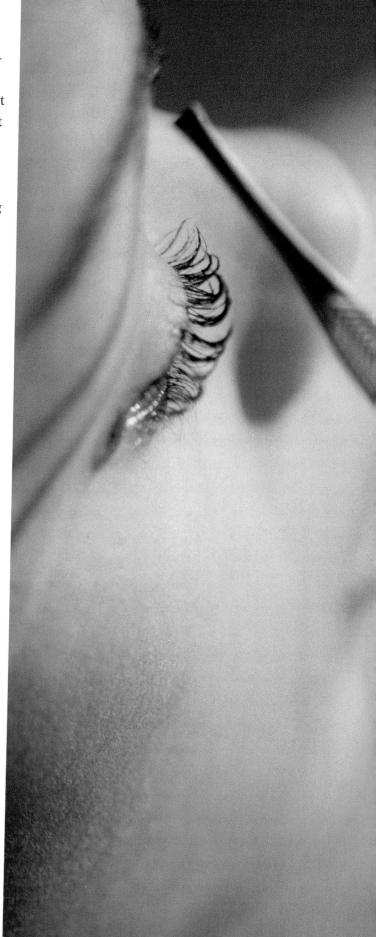

Check It Out

Now that the tweezing is finished, let's choose the right products for your brows. The most common eyebrow cosmetic is the pencil, which comes in a variety of colors for you to choose from. There are also finishing products for the brows such as gels and mousses. You will want to use a finishing formula that either dries clear or provides a transparent color that matches your brow pencil.

Color

You want to choose a pencil color that will naturally fill in sparse brows. Blondes look best in a light brown, taupe, or blonde; redheads should stick with shades of auburn; and brunettes need deep brown or charcoal colors. Your color should be applied with feather-like strokes to shape your brow's natural arch. I use two different colored eye pencils. I begin with a blonde pencil, and then fill in slightly with a taupe color for a more natural-looking brow.

The Answer Is

The success of any eyebrow pencil is found in the way it applies. Is it easy or difficult to put on? Does it pull and tug at the skin, or does it glide on smoothly? Does it stay on, or does it wear off before the end of the day? You should ask these questions when deciding on the right product.

The other items we need to evaluate are eyebrow gels, creams, and mousses. These products give your brows a well-groomed appearance. They can be worn alone or put on after you've applied the eyebrow pencil.

> **Gel**—Both conditioning and nonconditioning gels act like hairspray for unruly brows, holding them in place.
> **Cream or Mousse**—These products are usually available in a tube. They go on white but dry clear.
> **Clear Mascara**—Clear mascara comes in a conditioning gel that effectively grooms and sets brows without adding color.

Beauty Bonus

There is an alternative to tweezing unruly brows—giving them a good trim. Brows that are too long can look bushy, but if they are removed entirely they leave bare spots.

Brush your brows straight up and then use small manicure scissors to cut any hairs that are noticeably long. Cut hairs

Time Out with Tammy—

When I was growing up, no one was quite as makeup savvy as we are today. Our options were minimal compared to what you have at your fingertips. I didn't do much with my brows aside from tweezing them. I thought eyebrow pencils were only for gals who plucked off their brows and then drew them on with a pencil. Even then, that just didn't seem like the cool thing to do.

Unless you have no eyebrows or you've singed them off lighting the grill (I knew someone who did that), don't just pluck them out and draw them on!

Tammy's Tip • • • • • • • •
I use a clean mascara wand to brush my brows into shape. You can also use a soft bristled child's toothbrush as a substitute to costly eyebrow brushes.

one at a time and cut to various lengths so you don't end up with a blunt brow line. Be careful not to cut them too short. Once you're finished, brush them into place and follow through with any needed touch-ups.

How It Applies

Applying eyebrow pencil can be a little tricky at first. But you'll get the hang of it and be shading and shaping like a professional in no time.

#1: **Sharpen Pencil**—Always begin with a sharp pencil. You want your strokes to be thin, sharp, and precise. Some manufacturers offer self-sharpening pencils so you can avoid this step. Otherwise, include a sharpener in your purchase.

#2: **Feathery Strokes**—Start on the inside and work your way outward with light wispy strokes. Follow your natural brow line and carefully define its arch.

#3: **Pencil #2**—If you're using a second colored brow pencil, apply it in the same way you did the first color, but with less volume and intensity.

#4: **Grooming**—Set your brows with a gel, mousse, cream, or clear mascara. Using either a mascara wand or eyebrow brush, put a small amount onto the applicator and then brush it into place.

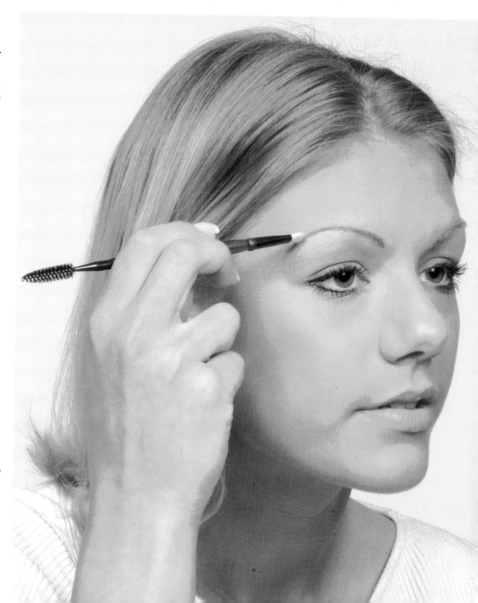

Tammy's Tip Use hair gel to set your brows. Just put a small amount on the applicator and brush into place.

Putting It to the Test

As you put eyebrow pencils, gels, and creams to the test, remember this important advice: If you apply too much eyebrow pencil, gently use a cotton swab to remove the excess. And if you make a mistake when you tweeze your brows, it will take them time to grow back. So be careful to pluck only one hair at a time, observing the results after each one you remove.

The key to eye-raising brows is in the arches.

Finding My Brow Products

Date: _____

Pencil Color #1

Product name:

Color:

Blends with brows without being too dark: YES / NO

Easy to Apply: YES / NO

Looks Natural: YES / NO

Pencil Color #2

Product name:

Color:

Blends well with pencil #1 resulting in a natural look: YES / NO

Easy to Apply: YES / NO

Looks Natural: YES / NO

Brow Gel, Cream, Mousse, or Clear Mascara

Product name:

Color:

Gives a natural well-groomed look: YES / NO

Easy to Apply: YES / NO

Looks Natural: YES / NO

My Perfect Match

Product Name:

Type of Brush:

Manufacturer's Name:

Beautiful brows bring shape and definition to your face. Their natural arch adds heightened splendor to your eye area. Unfortunately, well-maintained eyebrows don't come naturally. There always seem to be pesky hairs growing outside the brow line. In a continual effort to be outwardly beautiful, you must resort to a painful process of tweezing and waxing those unruly stray hairs.

The same is true of your inner beauty. Browse your mind. Continual reshaping of your thoughts is necessary in order to pluck sin from your life and live a balanced Christian life. Like your brows, this process takes constant upkeep on your part, but with a little ingenuity and know-how you can stay on top of it.

Brow-raising results begin with plucking sin from our lives.

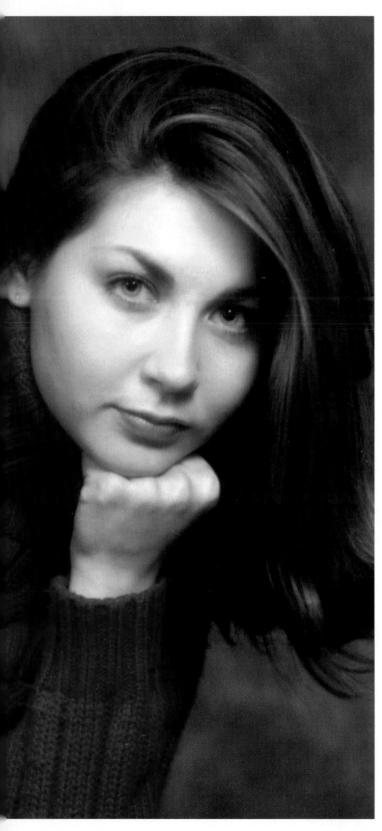

All of us need inspections to see if parts of our lives are growing outside the line of God's perimeters. We need to scrutinize the friends we make, the boyfriends we have, the music we listen to, and the extracurricular activities we join. In some circumstances, we need to pluck things from our lives that are causing us to sin.

Brow-Raising Facts

Think about it. Do you have friends that lead you astray? Does your boyfriend expect more than you should give? Does the music you listen to fill your mind with sex and drugs? Are your extracurricular activities an excuse for poor behavior?

Controlling your actions and defining your weaknesses takes a conscious effort on your part. You need to think before you act in order to tweeze out the negative and accentuate the positive areas of your life. By thinking these things through, you will understand yourself better.

Our everyday decisions affect who we are. Let's say you're dating a really awesome guy. You have to decide how you're going to spend your time together. Will you spend it alone or in a group setting? You decide to spend time alone, which leads to kissing, and then to petting, and eventually to having sex. You never planned on having sex— but you never planned *not* to either. If you had thought things through first, you would have contemplated the danger of being alone together. You would have chosen to nurture your relationship within the perimeters of group activities and public settings. This would have removed many sexual pressures in dating so you could relax and enjoy getting to know one another. I'm not saying you should play Monopoly with your parents, but you could go out to eat, bowling, or skating. You have options, and you're in control when you think first.

Plan ahead so you have a plan of action. Don't be overwhelmed with the thought that it's too hard. It's even harder to deal with the consequences of flirting with sin. Stay alert and think through your alternatives. Just like outer beauty, sin can be attractive on the surface. But don't be fooled. If you have to deal with sin's destructive core, you'll find out how ugly it really is.

When you play with fire, you will get burned. First-degree burns hurt, but, with a little nursing, leave no permanent scars. Second-degree burns cause excruciating pain and require specialized treatment to avoid infection. They leave scarring, but over the course of time the scars will fade and sometimes disappear. Third-degree burns are the most serious, destroying the nerve endings and leaving you numb to

Time Out with Tammy—

This story hits home with me every time I think back to it. At the time it occurred I thought it was sad, but I couldn't identify with the big picture because I had no experience as a mother. Back then I only felt the stinging embarrassment of my friend's mistake. It all started with her decision to go to a party. Everyone from school was there so her decision was easy; either go or be a nerd. So Carrie went. It was a great party; everyone was drinking and having the time of their lives.

However, a couple months later Carrie's good times turned into her worst nightmare. She got really sick, went to the doctor, and was told she was pregnant. She sat in the doctor's office in disbelief, not knowing how or when it could have happened. But then she remembered the party and being so wasted that she didn't even know how she'd gotten home. At the time she thought it was funny. She tried to recall somebody, anybody, but no one came to mind. She asked a couple of friends if they had seen her with anyone that night, and to her shame she was given several different names. She confronted each one of them, and they all denied knowing her sexually.

She was so alone, even her parents would have nothing to do with her. She contemplated an abortion but couldn't go through with it. She was going to suffer the humiliation of her consequences as she gained weight, developed stretch marks, wore maternity clothes, and obtained the title of unwed teenage mom. With her label came the question, "How would she care for a baby?" After all, she had no support from her family or the baby's father, whom she didn't even know.

On what should have been a joyous occasion, Carrie faced the darkest day of her life. She gave birth to a beautiful son that she held only once before the nurse whisked him away and delivered him to the adoptive parents. That brief moment when Carrie nuzzled the infant close to her heart is seared in her memory. She still wonders what became of her baby boy.

More than twenty years later, Carrie wishes she could go back and undo that one fateful decision to attend the party. Just a few hours of pleasure have left her with a lifetime of consequences. Sin leaves deep scars and ruins lives.

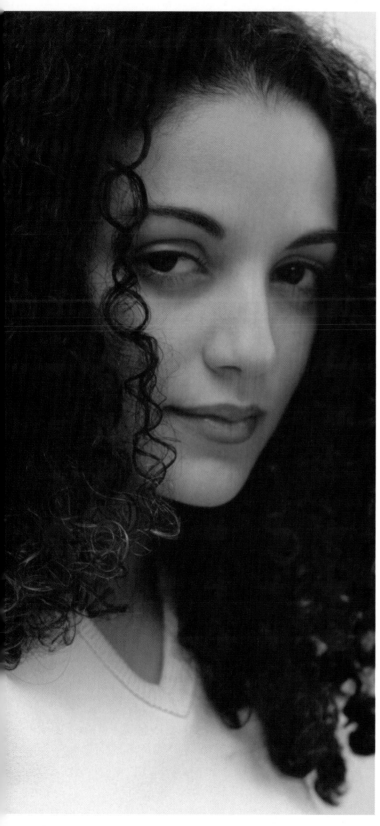

the pain and the severity of the burn. The scarring is extensive, and medical treatment and recovery can take weeks, months, or even years. In fact, some burns are so severe they ruin your life.

Play with sin and you will get burned. First-degree sin hurts but, with a little nursing, will heal and hopefully, like a child touching a hot stove, teach you a lesson about playing with fire. Second-degree sin causes excruciating hurt and requires specialized attention so it doesn't infect other areas of your life. Its scars are seared into your memory, but with time they will fade. Third-degree sin is the most serious. You've been involved long enough for it to make you numb to its damaging effects. The scarring is extensive, and rehabilitation can take weeks, months, or years. In fact, in some cases playing with sin ruins your life.

I hear heartbreaking stories like Carrie's repeated again and again by young girls just like you, and they always say the same thing: "If only I'd known . . .", "I didn't think . . .", "Why didn't I listen?"

Well girls, it's time to wake up and get smarter about making decisions. You need to listen to the advice of girls who have learned lessons the hard way. This is what I've heard them say: "There are consequences to your decisions because every action has a reaction." "Bad things can happen to you whether you think they can or not." "People can talk to you until they're blue in the face or write great books on the subject, but it's up to you to listen!"

I want to help you put out the fires of sin before you get burned. Like a spark that ignites a fire, our decisions can ignite sin. My goal is to make you stop and think, think, think! I wish I could sit down, look into your eyes, and scream the importance of what I'm saying before it's too late. I don't want you to end up another sad statistic.

Check It Out

Romans 12:2 (MESSAGE)—Don't become so well-adjusted to your culture that you fit into it without even thinking. Instead, fix your attention on God. You'll be changed from the inside out. Readily recognize what he wants from you, and quickly respond to it. Unlike the culture around you, always dragging you down to its level of immaturity, God brings the best out of you, develops well-formed maturity in you.

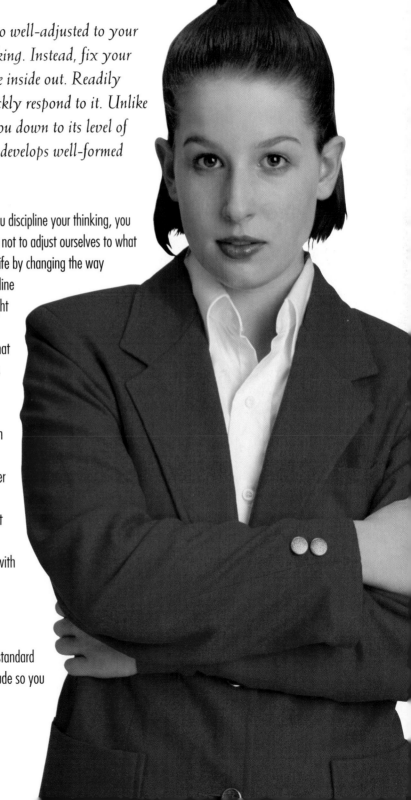

What we do is directly related to the way we think. If you discipline your thinking, you will control who you are and what you do. The Bible tells us not to adjust ourselves to what the people of this world are doing, but to start a fresh new life by changing the way we think as children of God. When you get your thinking in line with God's, you'll know what is good and pleasing in his sight and what he wants for you.

Consider this: You're the child of the Most High King. That makes you royalty. Do you think the princes and princesses of this world think the same way we do? Of course they don't. They've been conditioned to think differently, and that makes them behave differently. Ordinary tasks take on a whole new meaning for Prince William, for all eyes scrutinize his every move. Guess what? You're the daughter of the King of Kings, and those who are not heirs to the throne of God monitor everything about you. You might not have the paparazzi chasing you down, but non-Christians keep a watchful eye on your every move. And just as it is with Prince William, they delight when you mess up.

The Answer Is

So now that you know you've been called to a higher standard of living, how can you renew your mind, actions, and attitude so you can renew your surroundings?

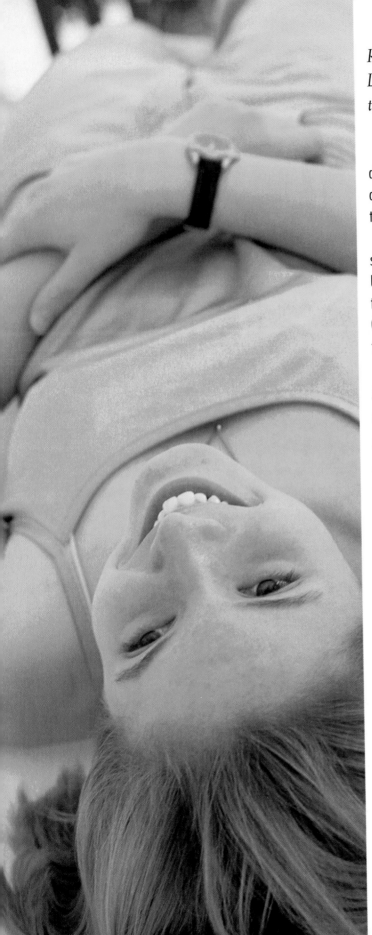

Romans 13:14—Clothe yourselves with the Lord Jesus Christ, and do not think about how to gratify the desires of the sinful nature.

This particular verse encourages us to be consistent in our daily Christ-like living. Every single morning we need to jump out of bed and dress ourselves in Christ. When we're clothed in his thoughts, we won't listen to our sinful nature.

If only it were that easy! Don't you wish you could grab something off the clothes rack to make you Christ-like? Unfortunately, you can't. It takes a conscious effort to master the art of thinking. But don't let that discourage you, because God has provided the know-how you need to master your thoughts.

Philippians 4:8 (NKJV)—Finally, brethren, whatever things are true, whatever things are noble, whatever things are just, whatever things are pure, whatever things are lovely, whatever things are of good report, if there is any virtue and if there is anything praiseworthy— meditate on these things.

Wow! What an awesome place to begin. If you meditate on everything listed in Philippians 4:8, you won't have time to think about anything else. You'll be so absorbed in the things of God that sin will have no place in your life.

Can you imagine dressing your mind in this fashion? First, start by clothing your mind in truth and adorning yourself with a noble outlook. Having a noble outlook makes you act like the royal princess you are. Next, accessorize your intellect with just, pure, lovely information that is of good report. Then tailor the outfit with virtue and praiseworthy thoughts.

Whatever things are true—Learn to recognize the truth in all situations and eliminate false beliefs.

Sometimes we want the wrong things to be true. Take Carrie's situation for example; she wanted so desperately to be popular that she convinced herself nothing was wrong with a little partying. But that was the furthest thing from the truth!

Whatever things are noble—Commit yourself to high moral standards, despite what others may think. The teasing is a small price to pay in comparison to the consequences of sinful standards.

Whatever things are just—Make fair decisions. Be fair to yourself and to others.

Whatever things are pure—Be authentic. Honesty and openness will keep you from making foolish mistakes.

Whatever things are lovely—Think beautiful! Don't think ugly thoughts about people. Look for the good in everyone.

Whatever things are of good report—Be a glass-is-half-full kind of person. Make a conscious effort to report the good news about others. People like to be around positive thinkers and encouragers.

If there is any virtue—Be a person of excellent character and integrity. Do the right thing even when no one else is watching except God.

If there is anything praiseworthy—First and foremost, God loves your praise for him. Be in mindful worship for all the great things he does for you. Second, praise other people too. Don't be stingy with compliments; use them often.

Meditate on these things—Get a new attitude by renewing your mind. You'll change your outlook and outfit yourself with fresh opinions, ideas, and standards. It's like changing your wardrobe; out with the old and in with the new!

Make a conscious effort to give each person in your immediate family one compliment a day.

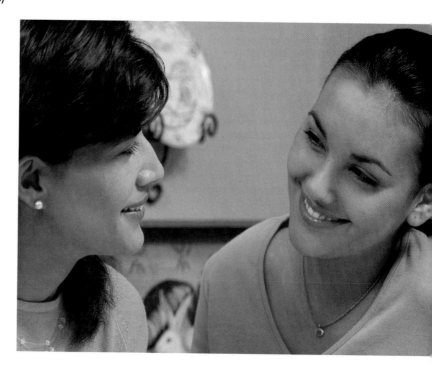

Beauty Bonus

Even though the Bible was written hundreds of years ago, it still applies to you today. It may seem doubtful, but it's true. Let's take a look at Philippians 4:8 in a practical manner. Let's say you've been cheating on your homework. How would Philippians 4:8 apply?

Whatever things are true—There's nothing truthful about cheating. Although you might be making the grade, the only one you're cheating is yourself. Be honest with yourself; study! And if studying means you only make a C+, at least you can be proud of yourself for earning it.

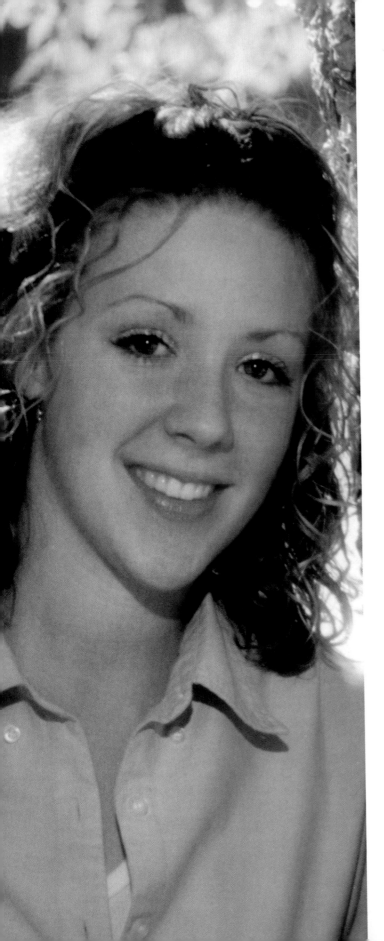

Whatever things are noble—Excellence in moral standards is much more important than excellent grades.

Whatever things are just—We demand fairness, so is it fair that you cheat?

Whatever things are pure—Honesty and openness will win a lot more friends than dishonesty and deceit. I struggled to make Cs and Ds in geometry, yet I knew a girl who was making As in the same class by cheating. She had very few friends because everyone knew she was a big cheat and a bigger phony.

Whatever things are lovely—There's nothing lovely about cheating. It makes you feel ugly inside. Your conscience can do a lot more damage to you than bad grades.

Whatever things are of good report—There won't be any good reports coming in on you when you're caught. You'll have to face your teachers, principal, and parents. This will make others doubt your credibility, giving them a negative attitude toward you.

If there is any virtue—Is the reputation of your character and integrity worth cheating even once to get a better grade? Your parents and teachers might not ever trust you again.

If there is anything praiseworthy—Study hard, do your best, and praise God for the ability to honestly get the grade you deserve. You'll feel worse when your parents and teacher praise you for receiving a grade you don't deserve.

Meditate on these things—If you think through the pros and cons of cheating, you'll see that even though you'll make the grade on your homework, you won't make the grade as a quality individual. It's too big of a risk to take. This one bad decision could affect not only the homework grade and the classroom grade, but it could scar your high school years permanently.

How It Applies

When you get down to it, there's only one way to pluck sin from your life and stay in line with God's perfect will, and that's with a changed mind. If you can change your eyebrows and do all the necessary maintenance in order to keep them looking great, then you can change your mind and do the necessary thinking to make you a great individual.

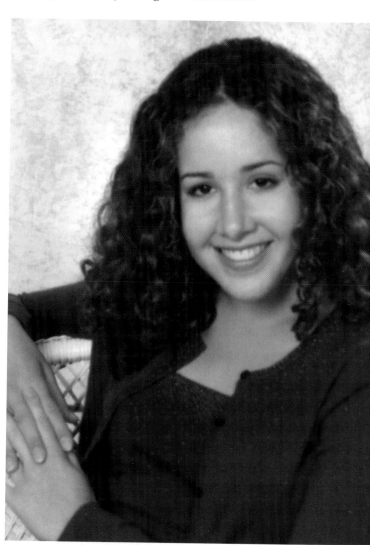

Galatians 6:7—Do not be deceived: God cannot be mocked. A man reaps what he sows.

Think things through. Know that there are reactions—good or bad—to your actions. Most important: remember that sin has consequences. Galatians 6:7 (MESSAGE) puts it this way, "No one makes a fool of God. What a person plants, he will harvest."

Putting It to the Test

Take a moment and think about struggles you're currently going through. How can you know what the right decision is? Find answers by putting it to the God test in Philippians 4:8.

Beauty Secret #8:
Reshape your brows and browse
your thoughts to renew
the "Super Model" in you.

Lips
Real Lip Service

Super moist, soft, smooth lips are something we all long for. Lips highlight our smiles, frame our words, and express our affection. We can even accessorize our wardrobe with the lip colors we wear. The possibilities are endless; we're only limited by our own creativity.

There are so many lip products available that I lost count when I was researching them for this book. There are products that primp, plump, or pop your lips with shape and color. The claims and costs listed on the wares are almost unbelievable, but don't panic. I've sorted through the hype and made some discoveries so that I can teach you how to be a lip expert in no time.

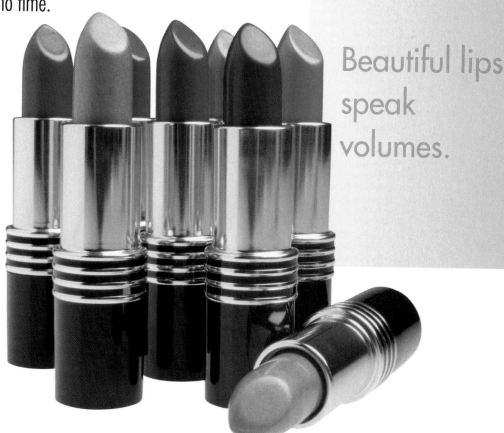

Beautiful lips speak volumes.

129

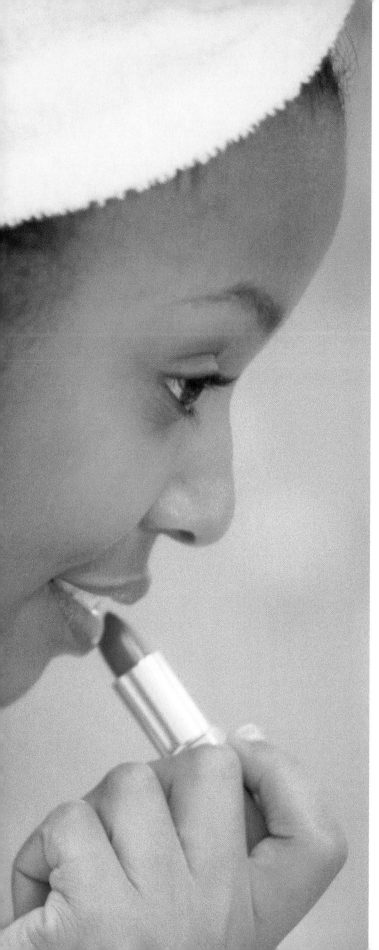

With so many lip products on the market it's hard to know where to begin. We'll start with the basics. Lip products define, express, and shield your lips. Lip liner gives definition to lips of all shapes and sizes; lipstick expresses your mood, creativity, and style; and lip balm, cream, and gloss contain rich emollients that prevent your lips from drying out. Sound overwhelming? It won't in a moment—keep reading.

Lip Sticking Facts

I have a drawer full of lip colors in every shade and variety from satin pink to sheer poppy, matte mocha, and fruity frost. It's all there, some of it for years. I even have mood lipstick that turns purplish green every time I put it on! Every now and then I clean them out and ask myself, "What ever possessed me to buy that color?"

Buying off-the-wall lip colors for special events is fun even though you may only wear them once, but buying colors on a whim is a whole different story. Why waste money on something you'll never wear when you can be a lip genius and buy the right stuff from the start?

You can eliminate extraneous buying by learning four basic principles: lip shape, type, texture, and color tones.

Check It Out

Let's start by defining the shape of your lips. Are they frowny, flat, full, imprecise, thin, or uneven?

What shape are your lips?

Frowny	**Flat**	**Full**	**Imprecise**	**Thin**	**Uneven**
Turned down corners	Little fullness	Too full	Faded lip line	Slender	Unbalanced

The Answer Is

Now that you know the shape of your lips, let's look at type, texture, and tone. To have great-looking lips you will need to learn what type of applicator will work best for you, what texture accentuates the shape of your lips, and what color tone will give you the look you want.

Type

There are two types of products you'll need for your lips: a lip pencil outlines and defines your lips and lip color fills them in. Lip liners come in two standard varieties—pencils you sharpen with a sharpener and twist type pencils that sharpen themselves. Lip color, on the other hand, comes in a variety of packaging.

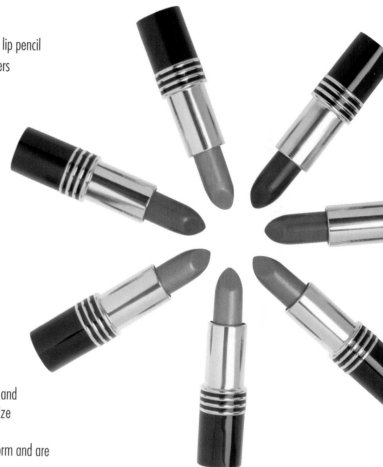

- **Lip Liner/Pencil:** Lip liner is used to define and shape lips of all types. Its opaque finish stays on and keeps your lip color from bleeding.
- **Lipstick Tubes:** Lipstick tubes are common and come in the widest range of textures and colors. They may be applied directly to the lips or with a lip brush.
- **Slim Line Sticks:** These skinny tubes of lipstick are designed for convenience. They come in a variety of texture and colors and may be applied directly to the lips or with a lip brush.
- **Chunky Lip Pencils:** Chunky lip pencils apply easily and give medium to full coverage but require a special size pencil sharpener.
- **Wand Applicator:** Wand applicators come in tube form and are typically only available in sheer or glossy finishes.
- **Lip Crème:** Lip crèmes come in tiny jars. They give medium to full coverage and must be applied with a lip brush or your finger.
- **Lip Balm:** Lip balms go on clear and are very waxy. They are formulated to heal and protect dry chapped lips.

Texture

Lip color comes in several textures. The formula you choose depends on the look you want to achieve and the shape of your lips. You can select matte, satin, frost, gloss, sheer, or clear finishes. On the next page you'll find a brief description of each kind and how it works.

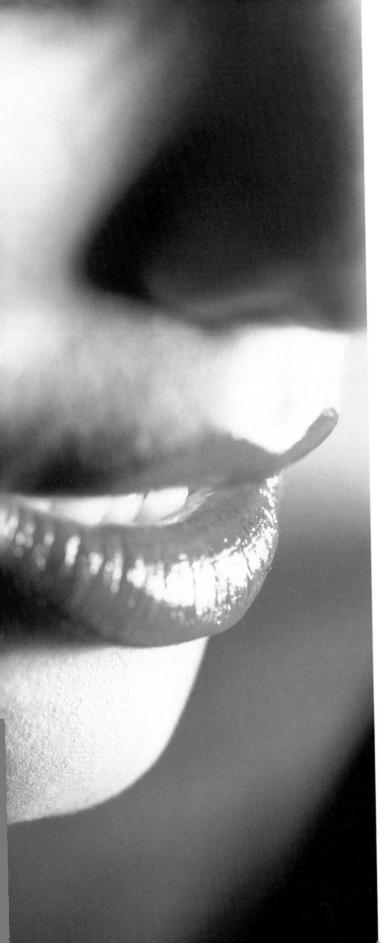

Matte Finish: Matte finishes give full intense coverage. They can be a little difficult to apply because they contain less oil than other textures.

Satin Finish: Satin finishes give medium to full coverage. They leave your lips feeling smooth and creamy with a touch of shine.

Frost Finish: Frost finishes give light to medium coverage. They give your lips ultra shimmer.

Gloss Finish: Gloss finishes go on shiny and sheer and come in many flavors, but they wear off easily. They can also cause lip color to bleed when applied on top of other colors.

Sheer Finish: Sheer finishes give lips natural translucent color with a little bit of shine.

Clear Finish: Clear finishes moisten lips with a natural wet shiny finish. Many clear finishes condition lips with a vitamin E complex.

Semipermanent Finish: Semipermanent finishes come in two-step formulas. Step one involves applying the lip color and allowing it to dry. Step two involves applying the protective top coat. During the course of the day you need only reapply the top coat (petroleum jelly may be substituted).

Color Tone

You'll find a bazillion different lip colors on the market, and what you don't find you can create yourself by mixing shades. You can buy stencils to paint on stars or hearts for a whimsical flair. Or you can go two-tone; using different colors on the upper and lower lips. The possibilities are endless.

Beauty Bonus

Some lip products contain added ingredients that are therapy to your lips. On the following page you'll find a list of these ingredients and what they'll do for you.

SPF (Sun Protection Factor): Lipstick and lip balms that contain SPF of 15 or higher combat the negative effects of the sun's harmful rays.

Vitamin E: Vitamin E oil moisturizes, softens, and smoothes dry, chapped lips.

Vitamin A: Vitamin A is a good emollient for reducing dryness and nourishing cell development.

Vitamin C: Vitamin C reduces skin irritation due to the sun's harmful UV rays. It may also produce collagen.

Collagen: Collagen applied to the surface of the lips helps repair damage by building scar tissue.

Tammy's Tip • • • • • • • • • • • • • • • •
Spread a thin layer of petroleum jelly on your lips before you go to bed. It seals in moisture and softens as you sleep, so you wake up with silky lips.

How It Applies

The key to great-looking lips is learning how to reshape them. Products with the correct combination of type, texture, and tone will turn up the corners on frowny lips, bring fullness to flat lips, minimize full lips, define imprecise lips, broaden thin lips, and balance uneven lips.

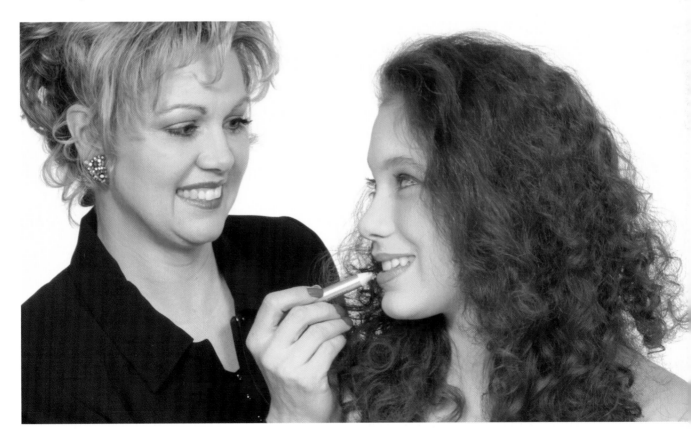

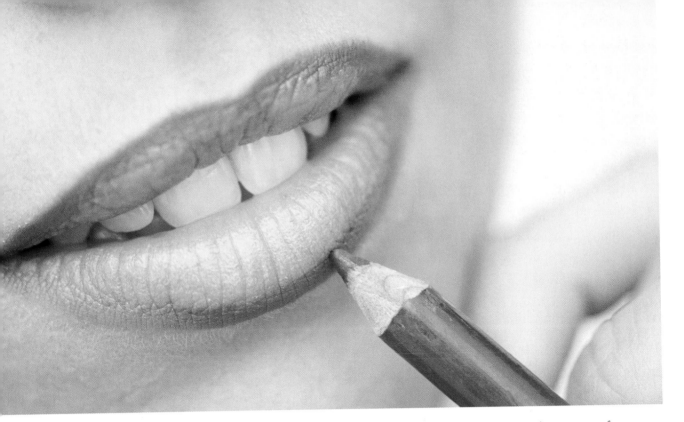

Frowny Lips: To reshape frowny lips you must redirect the downturned corners of your mouth. Using a lip liner, line your natural lower lip line first, slightly altering the corners upward. Next, line your natural upper lip line, joining the lines at the corners of your mouth. Use a lip brush and fill in with your choice of lip color and texture.

Flat Lips: To reshape flat lips you need to create the illusion of fullness. Line the outer edge of your natural lip line on both the top and bottom. Then use a lip brush and fill in with shiny lip color. Finish lips with a dab of gloss in the center of the lower lip. Stay away from matte finishes—they don't add dimension and fullness to your lips.

Full Lips: To reshape full lips you must visually minimize the lip area. Using a lip liner, line the inner edge of your natural lip line on both the top and bottom. Use a lip brush and fill in with a matte lip color. Stay away from glosses, as they will make your lips appear fuller.

Imprecise Lips: To reshape imprecise lips you must visually create a lip line. Using a liner, draw in the V shape on your upper lip. Next, extend the line outward to the corners following your natural lip line. Line your lower lip following your natural lip line. Then use a lip brush to fill in with a matte color. Stay away from glosses—they can blur the definition of your lip liner.

Tammy's Tip • • • • • • • • • • •
Always keep your lip liner sharpened to a fine point to ensure a precise line.

134

Thin Lips: To reshape thin lips you must create the illusion of fullness. Using a lip liner, line the outer edge of your natural lip line on both your upper and lower lips. Use a lip brush and fill in with satin, sheer, or glossy lip color. Stay away from dark colors, because they make your lips look smaller.

Uneven Lips: To reshape uneven lips you must create balance by redefining the borders of your lips. Line the inner edge of your natural lip line on the thicker part of your lips and line the outer edge of your natural lip line on the thinner part of your lips. Next use a lip brush and fill in with a satin lip color.

Putting It to the Test

Lip color is fun. It's the one cosmetic you can use to make radical or subtle changes to your look. Have fun experimenting with all the colors of the rainbow, and remember that if you don't like it, it's easily removed without messing up the rest of your makeup. When you smile at someone it's contagious, and they usually smile back. So smile in style!

The key to good-looking lips is in the smile.

Finding My Lip Products

Date: _____

Lip Liner Color

Product name:

Color:

Easy to Apply: YES / NO

Too Light: YES / NO

Too Dark: YES / NO

Lip Colors

Product name:

Color:

Texture:

Product name:

Color:

Texture:

Product name:

Color:

Texture:

My Perfect Match

Product Name:

Color Tone:

Type:

Manufacturer's Name:

Flattering lips are one of our most expressive qualities. The lip color we choose adds a subtle or strong change to our overall look. It's the one cosmetic we're never caught without. We tote it with us wherever we go so we can touch up and reapply as needed.

But even though we're often ready with a tube of lipstick, we sometimes forget a very important necessity—a mirror. Even experts need a mirror to apply their lip color with no mistakes. Reflection is key. It's important when we apply makeup to our lips and even more important as we make up the words we speak. You may have gorgeous lips, but if you don't think before you speak, they get ugly really quickly. Their size, shape, and color do not compare with their power, impact, and influence.

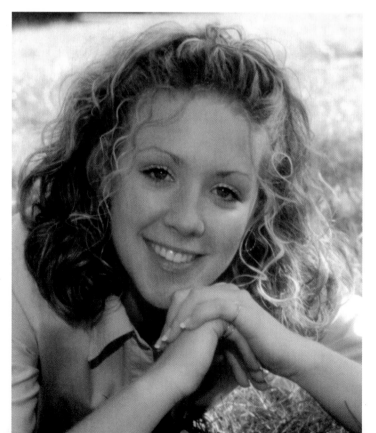

Lip sticking words begin with reflecting on what we say before we say it.

Did you ever stop to think about how something seemingly so small in comparison to the rest of your body can get you into so much trouble? "Me and my *big* mouth!" An important thing to learn about lips is how to carefully choose the words that come out of them. After all, the words that come off our lips are much more important than what we put on them.

Lip Sticking Facts

Words hurt. Remember the children's rhyme, "Sticks and stones may break my bones but names can never hurt me"? I used that rhyme all the time as a kid to protect myself from being hurt by mean words. In reality, broken bones will heal in six weeks but name-calling leaves scars that can last a lifetime.

Check It Out

The Bible speaks volumes about the words we say, which could only mean one thing: this must be one super important topic. Consider James 3:2–10. This passage is a lot to take in all at once, so we're going to look at it a little at a time.

James 3:2—We all stumble in many ways. If anyone is never at fault in what he says, he is a perfect man, able to keep his whole body in check.

James tells us if we could find someone who speaks the perfect words, we'd find a person in control of his or her life. Do you know anyone like that? I don't. But I do know people who have learned to have better control over life. Think about it. If we could learn to control our words, then we could learn to control our actions too. But if we have no control over our tongues, then we have no control over the rest of ourselves either.

James 3:3-5a—When we put bits into the mouths of horses to make them obey us, we can turn the whole animal. Or take ships as an example. Although they are so large and are driven by strong winds, they are steered by a very small rudder wherever the pilot wants to go. Likewise the tongue is a small part of the body, but it makes great boasts.

Time-Out
with Tammy—

My relationship with my sister is a prime example of the permanent scars that words leave between two people. In grade school, junior high, and high school, we fought and argued *worse* than cats and dogs. The things we said to one another should never be said to anyone, let alone a sibling you love. As adults those words ended in years of silence before time finally healed the hurt.

Now you may be thinking, "I'd be thrilled if I never heard from my sister or brother again," but that's not true. You would miss the good times and wish there were more of them. My sister and I live on opposite coasts now and regret not being closer geographically and relationally. We cherish getting together every few years at Christmas and talking occasionally on the phone. Don't let this happen to you. Learn to control your tongue before it's too late. You can never take back words or gain lost time.

I'd like to end this time out by saying one thing: "Lisa I'm (still) sorry, and I love you."

Is there anyone who needs to hear those words from you before it's too late?

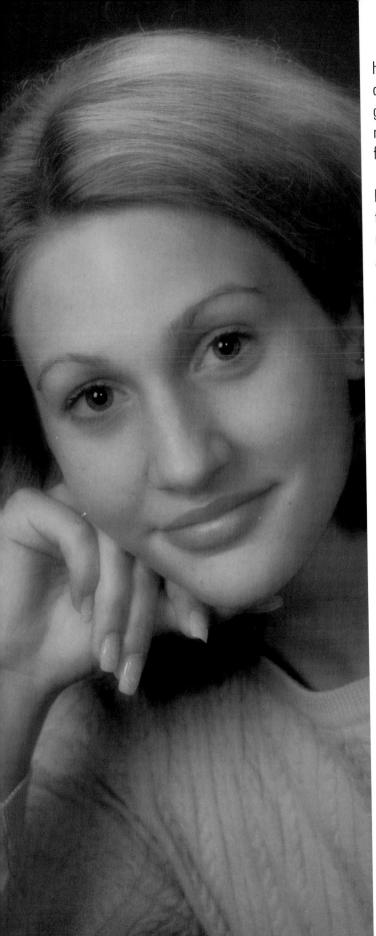

Have you ever stood next to a full-grown horse? The average height of a horse is fifteen hands tall and the average weight is one thousand pounds. That's a lot of weight to control, especially given that it has it's own mind and will. Yet you can control every movement of a one-thousand-pound horse with a twelve- to fourteen-ounce bit, less than one percent of its body weight!

And I won't even venture to guess how much a ship weighs but I have traveled on a cruise ship that contained several decks, two swimming pools, three stage theaters, a mini shopping mall, and nine restaurants. It was like a massive floating city! And yet when you compare the enormity of the ship to the tiny rudder that steers its movement, it seems almost inconceivable that something so small has so much power and influence.

You might be asking yourself what on earth a horse and a ship have to do with your tongue. Well, a bit in comparison to a horse seems miniscule, a rudder compared to the size of a ship seems insignificant, and your tongue measured against the rest of your body mass seems tiny. But in all three cases these teeny objects seize control. In simple terms, your tongue controls you if you don't control your tongue!

James 3:5b-6—Consider what a great forest is set on fire by a small spark. The tongue also is a fire, a world of evil among the parts of the body. It corrupts the whole person, sets the whole course of his life on fire, and is itself set on fire by hell.

One spark can turn into an uncontrollable forest fire, destroying thousands of acres of trees. Your tongue works like that spark through slander and gossip. And just like a forest fire, it usually happens by accident. You don't mean to hurt anyone, but you feel like a big shot at the time, giving details that everyone wants to know about your friend. But then your friend finds out you revealed her secrets and confronts you about it. You lie to cover up what you did, but it's too late. She feels hurt and her reputation is ruined. Your friendship is over and you're not feeling so big anymore, but rather small.

Gossip and backbiting can be girls' biggest problems. Inquiring minds want to know things, and we're too willing to tell—and if we *don't* know, we're often willing to make it up as we go. Your tongue can be your greatest enemy. Don't let it start a fire you can't control.

James 3:7–8—All kinds of animals, birds, reptiles and creatures of the sea are being tamed and have been tamed by man, but no man can tame the tongue. It is a restless evil, full of deadly poison.

What a scary thought: You could tame a lion before you could tame your own lying tongue, or you could charm a poisonous cobra more easily than controlling the poison that comes from your own lips. Does this sound a little outrageous? Then think about this. Let's say you get a new puppy and you have to train it. In my past experience it's taken me four to six weeks to train a puppy, and it required lots of time, effort, consistency, and positive reinforcement. Training your tongue requires the same things. Take time out to think before you speak, giving careful consideration to how the end results are going to affect you and others. Make a conscious effort to consistently discipline your mouth. And when you offend or lie, be responsible, apologize, and tell the truth. Finally, positively reinforce your mind with Bible verses and prayer so the first words out of your mouth aren't curse words or expressions that use the Lord's name in vain. Like a puppy, training your tongue may seem hopeless at times. There will still be accidents to clean up after, but the end results are well worth the battle.

James 3:9–10—With the tongue we praise our Lord and Father, and with it we curse men, who have been made in God's likeness. Out of the same mouth come praise and cursing. My brothers, this should not be.

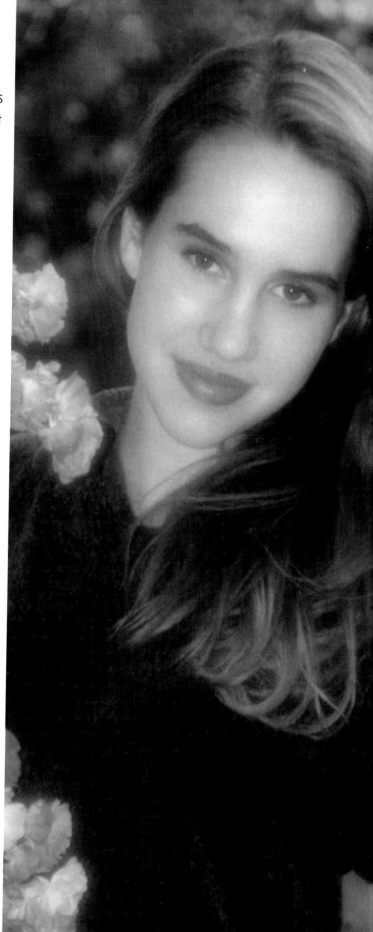

This is grand finale of this passage. The lips that we lie, gossip, slander, curse, and manipulate with are the same lips we praise, worship, glorify, magnify, and exalt God with. Girlfriends, this shouldn't be so!

Are you starting to see the big picture? Our little lips have big control, not only over what we say and do, but also over who we are as individuals. When you get your lips under control, you'll become utterly beautiful.

The Answer Is

The key to safeguarding your tongue can be found in your **L.I.P.S.**
   L—Listen to what you're going to say before you say it. Think before you speak.
   I—Improve your vocabulary. If you really want to impress people, learn new words.
   P—Pray for conscious awareness in all you say and do. Ask God for discernment.
   S—Speak two positives for every negative you say. Be encouraging, not discouraging.

Psalm 141:3—Set a guard over my mouth, O Lord; keep watch over the door of my lips.

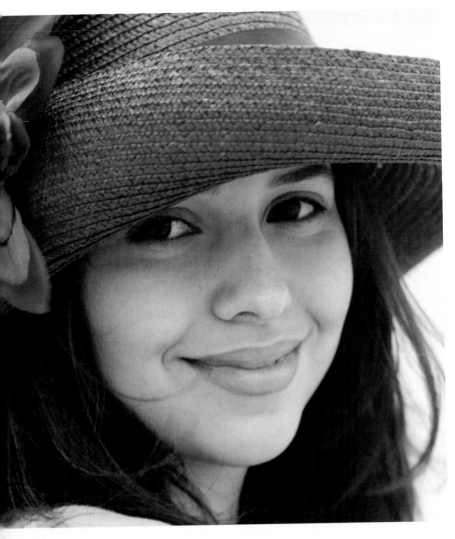

Beauty Bonus

Beautiful lips express a mood, accentuate your makeup, and accessorize your wardrobe. They communicate a lot about you on the outside, but what about the inside? Do your lips emphasize an uplifting or condemning tone? Do they compliment talking with silence? And do they display warm affection or cold aversion?

Sometimes what we say isn't half as important as the way we say it. The tone we use dictates the mood of the conversation. For example:

"What should I wear?" (Inoffensive question)
"WHAT SHOULD I WEAR!" (Offensive statement)

I used that on more than one occasion with my mother, and when I'd get in trouble for talking to her in that tone, I'd innocently reply, "I only asked you what I should wear." Of course I knew it wasn't the comment I made, but the tone I used, that got me grounded. Be careful with the tone and sarcasm in your voice and you'll save yourself a lot of future grief and groundings.

Have you ever heard, "You have two ears and one mouth, which means you should listen twice as much as you talk"? I believe God created us this way purposefully. It's a good indicator that we need to be quiet and listen to what's going on around us. Sometimes we're so busy doing all the talking that we're insensitive to the needs of others. We need to deactivate our mouths and practice active listening skills like looking directly at the person who is talking and giving them our undivided attention without interrupting.

We also need to "listen" closely to what their body language is saying. Sometimes people only say half of what they want you to understand, but their body language will convey the rest. For instance, let's say your friend asks you, "Do you think Matthew is nice?" You might answer abruptly if you don't notice her body language. She's sort of looking down and drawing squiggles on the ground with her foot, indicating that she's really trying to say, "I like Matthew and I think he's a great guy, but I don't know how to get him to notice me." Be less

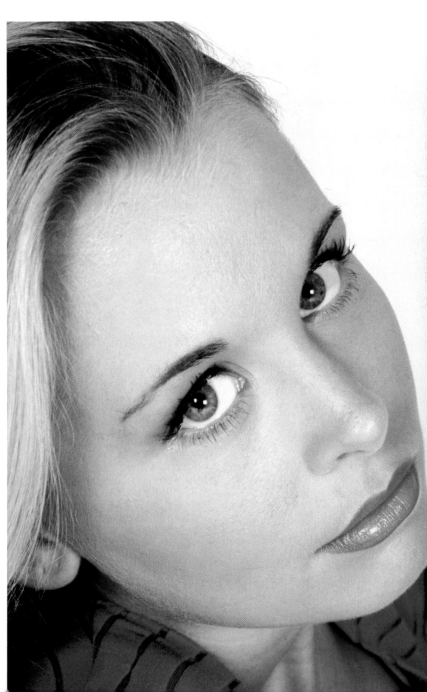

Tammy's Tip

Don't interrupt. Nothing you have to say is more important than listening. You gain respect by listening to what others are saying, not by talking so others will listen.

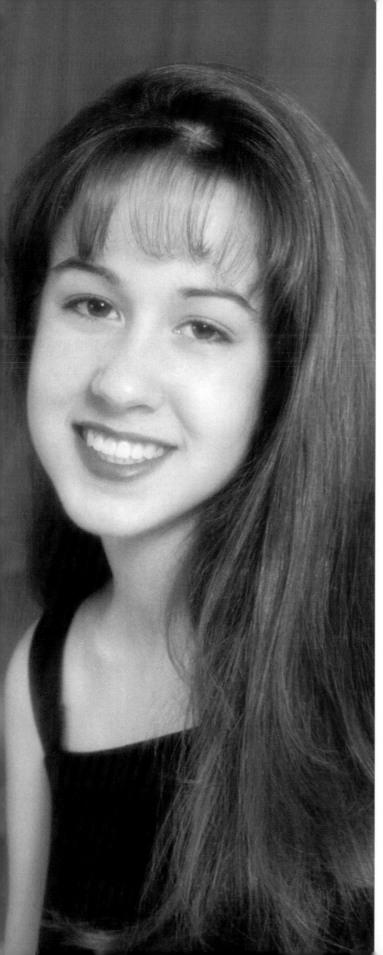

active in your talking and more active in your listening habits.

The last thing I want to talk to you about is affection or lack of it. From a mother's standpoint I can let you in on a little secret: I live for the moments when my kids give me a hug and kiss and tell me they love me. Displaying affection for the ones you love (and I'm not talking about making out with your boyfriend) fills that critical need for acceptance.

Do your parents ever say no to something you're desperate for? You beg to spend the night at your friend's house but your parents won't let you go, so you give them the silent treatment. You're determined to let them know how mad you are even if you have to avoid their attention for a solid week. Does it work? Not according to my past experience. From what I've encountered, you're much better off agreeing to disagree with them when you don't understand their decision. Be honest and tell them you don't get it but you'll respect and obey what they've decided. In turn you'll start gaining their trust as a responsible young adult. Don't let arguments stand in the way of affection. It's in the midst of the greatest hurt that the most healing can come from our lips in the words, "I love you" followed by a kiss on the cheek.

How It Applies

Applying positive communication to your lips takes a conscientious effort on your part. Reshape your conversation by controlling your tongue. Evaluate the type of words you use. Do they please God? What about the tone you use? Is it going to get you into trouble? Think before you speak.

When words aren't appropriate, apply texture to your lips by learning to be quiet. Practice good listening skills so you know the depth of the conversation even when very little is said. Listen twice as much as you talk.

And my favorite piece of advice: Give your mom a kiss and tell her you love her. Establish acceptance for one another by expressing affection in your relationships.

This might sound like a lot to apply all at once, but like the right type, tone, and texture of lip color, it will make a noticeable difference.

Putting It to the Test

Your lips say a lot about you. They can be your most flattering or unflattering feature depending on what you apply to them. Apply them with kindness and you will be kind. Apply them with encouragement and you will be encouraging. Apply them with wisdom and you will be wise. Apply them with compliments and you will be admired for your beautiful lips.

Beauty Secret #9: Define and shield the communication of your lips to express the "Super Model" in you.

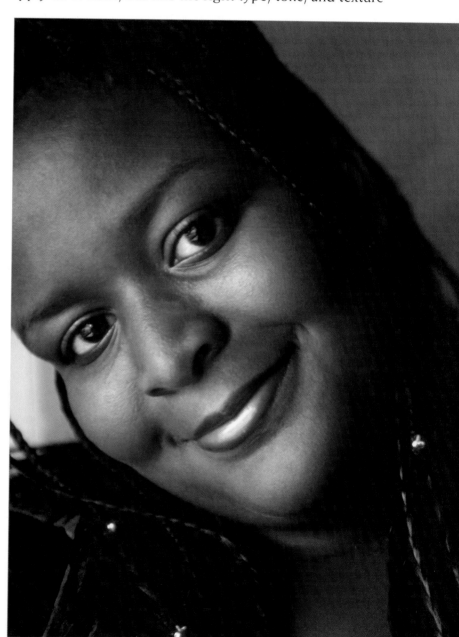

Powder

The Finished Product

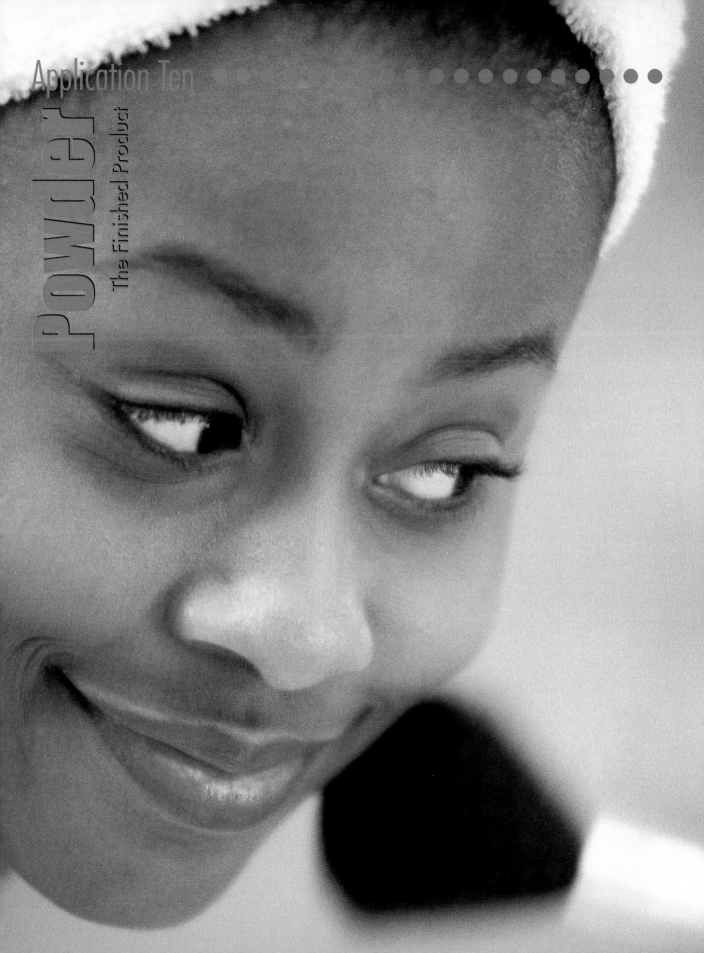

Powder is the final touch to a finished look. Just a light dusting sets your makeup in place, evens out your skin tone, and prevents oily breakthrough shine, leaving your complexion with a smooth and flawless appearance.

Like other cosmetics, powders come in many varieties. You can buy finishes ranging from iridescent loose powder to matte compacts. The choices abound, but with a little bit of know-how and a good powder brush you'll be a sweeping success!

The transparency of powder makes it a very useful cosmetic. It can be worn on bare skin to combat oily shine or dusted lightly over foundation to give your skin a smooth surface for the application of powdered blush. And if you apply too much blush, you can blend in a little powder and remedy that too! Powder is one cosmetic you don't want to be caught without.

Powder is the last step to a beautiful finish.

145

Loose Compact Facts

Powders come in two forms, loose or pressed. Loose powder is sold in small jar-like containers, and pressed powder comes in a solid form, pressed into a compact. Both are a great investment. I use loose powder in the mornings when applying my makeup and pressed powder throughout the day for on-the-go touch-ups.

Loose powder is blended into a fine lightweight texture that glides on easily with a powder brush, creating a professional-looking finish. Unfortunately, it may deposit powder onto your clothes too. You can easily solve this problem by draping a towel over you before you use powder.

Compact powders have a denser consistency and include a powder puff for quick application. The drawback is that they tend to look chalky unless they are well blended. To ensure natural-looking results, carry a portable makeup brush with you and gently sweep the chalky residue from your face. Portable makeup brushes come in a twist tube container and can be purchased at your local cosmetic counter.

As you can see, both of these products have advantages and disadvantages. But both are essential to producing a beautiful fresh-all-day look.

Check It Out

Like foundation, powders are sold in a wide range of colors and offer various types of coverage. To determine what kind of powder you should use, identify your skin's three Ts: type, texture, and tone. (Refer to the "Check It Out" section of application 2.) This basic knowledge will help you purchase powder with the right coverage and color for your skin.

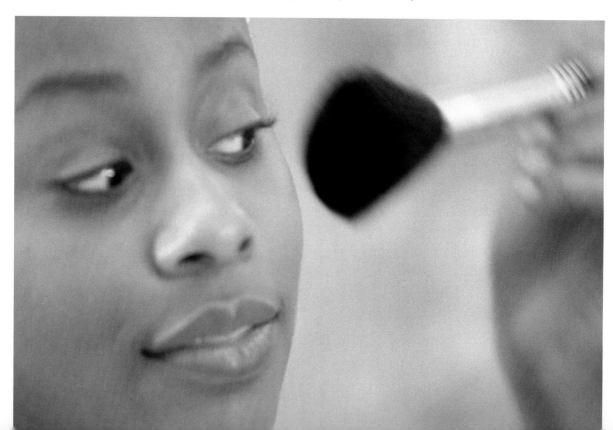

Coverage

Powders are formulated to offer various degrees of coverage for differing skin types. Some powders are designed to give a sheer transparent finish, while others offer a light-diffusing matte finish. Read the product label to know exactly what you're getting.

Color

Like other cosmetics, powders come in a wide range of colors. The only question is which one should you pick? To find a powder that matches your skin tone, use the same guidelines you did when choosing the right foundation. To make this process easy, many manufacturers have matched up the names of their foundations and powders.

The Answer Is

Even though powders only come in the form of loose or compact, there are still different formulas to pick from. Here's what to look for:

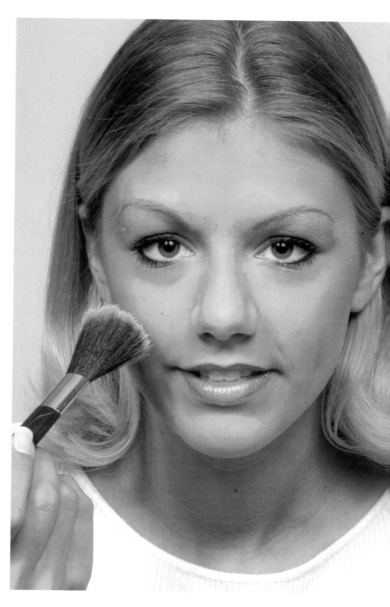

Matte Finish: Matte finish powders have a dense consistency that neutralizes skin discolorations and reduces oily shine. They can be worn alone or with foundation. Due to their heavy texture, they need to be applied lightly in order to avoid caking.

Sheer Finish: Powders with a sheer finish highlight the skin with a light reflective glaze of see-through color. It sets foundation and concealer and blends easily for lightweight coverage.

Translucent Finish: Translucent powders create a no-glow effect that perfectly sets makeup. It's best to lightly dust it across your face after you've applied your makeup, but before you apply your mascara so you don't dull your lashes.

Shimmer/Iridescent Finish: Shimmer or iridescent powder is a subtle way of adding a pearl-like sparkling finish to your cheekbones and shoulders. Avoid using it over your entire face.

Tammy's Tip
For suntanned skin, sweep your blush brush through your blusher and then a powder bronzer. Tap off the excess and then apply the two-in-one color to your cheeks.

147

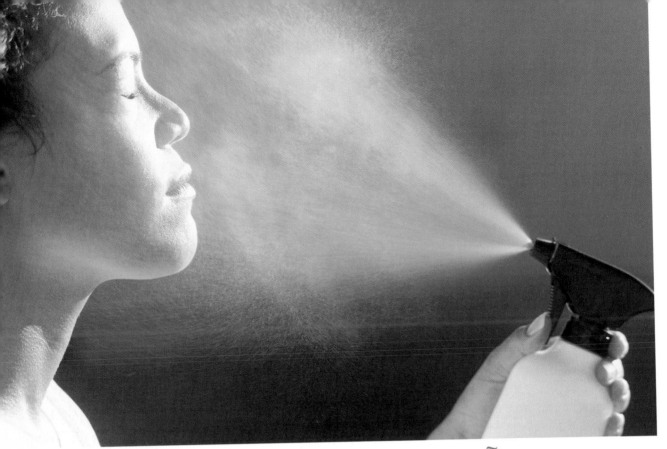

Bronze Finish: Bronzer is a great way to get that sun-kissed glow even when you haven't been out in the sun. Using a powder brush, dust it sparingly across your forehead, cheekbones, nose, and chin.

Tammy's Tip • • • • • • • • • •
I carry a small (trial size) spray bottle of purified water in my purse for on-the-go touch-ups.

Beauty Bonus

If breakthrough shine goes beyond average powder touch-ups, which are usually three to four times a day, then you may want to consider changing your moisturizer, foundation, or both. Your skin can change with the seasons or with hormones, so you may need to adapt your skin care and cosmetic products to meet its evolving needs.

How It Applies

Powder is the one cosmetic that can be applied before, during, or after you put on your makeup. Use the information below as a guide to help you determine which application will work best for you.

Before: Powder can be used in place of foundation. Apply it to clean bare skin to help combat shine and leave your face with a natural-looking matte finish. To apply, dip your powder brush in loose powder and then tap off the excess. Lightly dust it over your face, blending as you go to avoid caking. Touch up with a compact powder as needed.

During: After you've applied foundation and concealer, lightly dust your face with powder to set them in place. This will help keep your mascara from rubbing off when you blink your eyes, and it will create a smooth-textured surface so powdered blush will glide on evenly. To apply, dip your powder brush in loose powder and then tap off the excess. Lightly dust it over your face, blending as you go to avoid caking. Touch up with a compact powder as needed.

Helpful hint: For hard-to-conceal scars or blemishes, apply your foundation and then dab a little concealer over them. Lightly blend the outer edge into your foundation. Next, dip the tip of your makeup wedge into the powder and pat over the area, gently pressing the powder into the area to be concealed. Follow up by lightly dusting your face with powder as directed above.

After: Translucent powder creates a shine-controlling shield and sets

It was Julie's big day! She jumped out of bed, dressed in her new outfit, curled her hair, and applied her makeup a little heavier than usual. She gobbled down her breakfast and headed out the door for school. This was the day she'd represent her school in the locally televised state spelling bee. Upon her arrival at the school, she ran into Paul. Her day couldn't get any better than this. She'd had a crush on Paul for weeks but never had the nerve to go up and talk to him. Now he was approaching her! "Hi, Julie. You look really nice. I like your hair that way." Julie almost fainted right there on the spot but regained her composure and said, "Thanks. Today's the state spelling bee." "Oh yeah. I almost forgot," Paul replied. "Let me give you a hug for luck." Then Paul gave her a hug, turned, and walked away.

As Paul walked into his first class everyone started giggling. One of the guys yelled out, "Hey Paul, have a little trouble putting your makeup on this morning? Isn't it supposed to go on your face?" Paul looked down and there was Julie's makeup all over his white shirt. He turned red and tried to deliver his excuse, but there was no overcoming the razzing.

When Julie got back to school that day she raced up to Paul to share her second-place victory. She was quickly dejected when he said, "Just stay away from me and don't come near me again." If Julie had only set her makeup with translucent powder, Paul would have probably shared in her excitement. Instead, her heart was broken and her big day was ruined.

I've had this happen to me before, and I know it's no fun trying to get makeup out of garments. The oils from your face penetrate the fabric and the makeup soaks in, often leaving a stain. The best treatment is to have the garment dry cleaned immediately or make a detergent paste out of laundry stain remover and laundry detergent. Dampen the spot and spread this mixure on, rubbing it into the fabric. Allow it to set for an hour before you wash the garment in the washing machine.

your makeup into place. Dip your powder brush into loose translucent or sheer powder and then tap off the excess. Lightly dust it over your face, blending as you go to avoid caking. Touch up with a compact powder as needed.

Final Touch: The trick here is to powder your face without looking powdery. To avoid looking like you were attacked by a giant powder puff, gently dust off the excess with a powder brush (large puff brush) and then mist your face with an atomizer (misting spray bottle) filled with purified water. Blot gently with a tissue, paying close attention to the eyebrow area.

Putting It to the Test

Powder has a variety of uses. Not only does it set your makeup, correct blush bloopers, and control shine, it also makes your pores less visible and hides blemishes and scars, leaving your face with a silky smooth appearance. It's undoubtedly one of the best additions to your purse and cosmetic bag.

The key to a beautiful finish is in the powder.

Finding My Powder

Date: _____

Skin Type:

Skin Texture:

Skin Tone:

What type of coverage will you need:

   Matte   Sheer   Translucent

When will you apply powder?

   Before   During   After make up

In the spaces below write down the name of the product and the color you are testing. Determine if it matches your skin tone without caking or looking chalky.

Product name:

Color:

Does it match your skin tone/foundation? YES / NO

Is it the right amount of coverage? YES / NO

Product name:

Color:

Does it match your skin tone/foundation? YES / NO

Is it the right amount of coverage? YES / NO

Product name:

Color:

Does it match your skin tone/foundation? YES / NO

Is it the right amount of coverage? YES / NO

My Perfect Match

Product Name:

Color:

Manufacturer's Name:

Powder gives your face a fresh, flawless finish. Its fine consistency prevents makeup meltdown with a transparent shield of protection. Whether worn over foundation or alone, it leaves a sheer, see-through finish and improves the natural radiance of your skin.

Transparency is the defining issue here—it lets the *real* you shine through. No more phony business. It's all about being honest with yourself and others so you can develop true friendships and avoid superficial relationships.

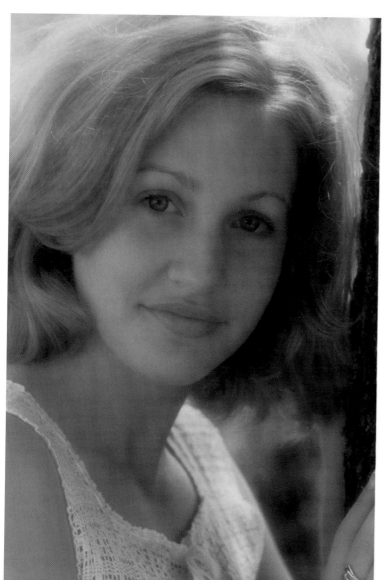

Transparency reveals the real you.

I can remember lying about something as ridiculous as where I bought a pair of shoes. A girl at school complimented my sneakers and asked where I got them. I was too embarrassed to tell her I bought them from a cheap discount store, so I told her that I bought them at an expensive department store. Sounds like a harmless lie, right? Wrong. My PE teacher was standing nearby and heard the whole conversation. She took it upon herself to embarrass me by saying, "Last night I saw those very same shoes at a discount store."

It was outlandish for me to think that I would be popular for shopping at an upscale department store, but I did. Instead, the gal told her group of friends and they delighted in making fun of me. I tried to avoid them throughout junior high and high school. Needless to say, we never became friends.

Being open and honest is one of the toughest things for teens to do. We're so afraid of what our friends might think that we often lie to gain acceptance. But when we act fake to gain popularity, we're not being accepted for who we really are.

True friendships are based on trust, which is developed by being transparent in your relationships. It's important to be real in every area of your life. Transparency is one character trait you'll never want to be caught without.

Fake-Out Facts

There are basically two factors that prevent us from being honest with others. One factor is our insecurities. We don't feel confident enough to let our guard down so others will get to know us; instead we hide behind lies and exaggerations, hoping for instant popularity. We lie to make ourselves look good, not realizing how bad we'll look when the truth comes out.

Short-sighted pride also keeps us from being real with others. Pride seems to affect us because we're too self-confident, but in reality it usually affects us because we're too insecure. Pride is a defense mechanism to make us feel good about ourselves, and it will take over every area of our lives if we let it. Pride leads to a narrow-minded (compact) attitude, generating a negative outlook toward others. But as you look down on others, they look down on you. It's a lose/lose combination that has destructive results if you don't get it under control.

Check It Out

Proverbs 16:18—Pride goes before destruction, a haughty spirit before a fall.

I love the book of Proverbs. It contains so much practical insight on day-to-day living. In fact, if you've ever thought about reading the Bible but didn't know where to begin, Proverbs is a great place to start. Take Proverbs 16:18 for example, which says pride comes before a fall. In other words, when your head swells you'll end up falling flat on your face. And from what I've experienced, the bigger the head, the harder the fall and the tougher the consequences.

I once met a gal who was an awesome soccer player. She was so good that many colleges were actively recruiting her. I went to watch one of Amanda's games and was quite impressed by her performance level but taken aback by her cocky attitude. From the bleachers I could see how much her teammates detested her arrogance and bossiness toward them.

Remember what Proverbs said? Pride comes before the fall. There were only a couple of minutes left in the game when Amanda tripped and lost control of the ball. The reaction of her teammates said it all; they laughed and scoffed at her. They didn't seem to care that the other team scored in the final seconds and won the game. They were rejoicing in Amanda's defeat. Even as she was exiting the field I overheard the coach sarcastically say, "It couldn't have happened to a nicer person."

When we got to the parking lot, Amanda began to cry. I put my arm around her shoulder and said, "Don't worry about it. Everyone has off days. You'll do better next time." She began to sob uncontrollably and replied, "It's not that. I don't have any friends. They all hate me." As we drove home I talked to her about her attitude and how it affected the team. At first she got defensive and said, "They're just jealous." As we continued talking, she began to realize that her pride was masking fear. She was afraid she wouldn't earn a soccer scholarship. And even though she was a top-notch player, she felt threatened by her teammates. In a desperate effort to protect her position, she began building herself up by tearing everyone else down. She had become so driven by fear that she didn't realize what she was doing until it was too late.

Now came the hard part; she would have to humble herself and accept the consequences of her pride. Amanda had lacked humility, a trait that is completely opposite of pride. Where pride is haughty, humility is humble, and where pride brings destruction, humility brings honor.

Proverbs 18:12—Before his downfall a man's heart is proud, but humility comes before honor.

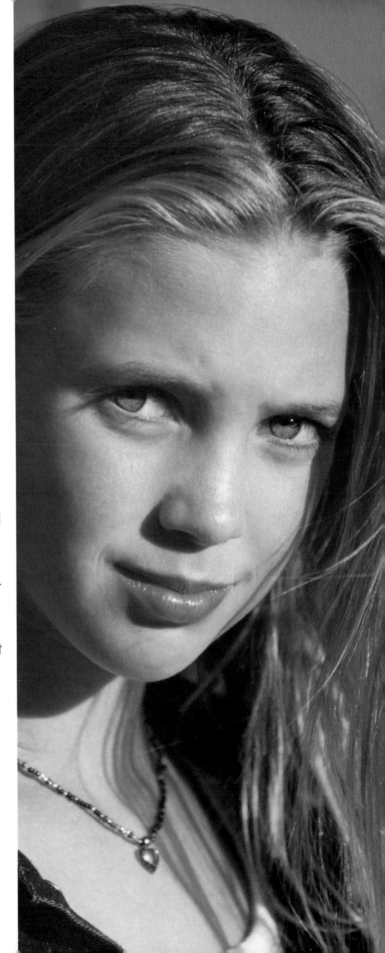

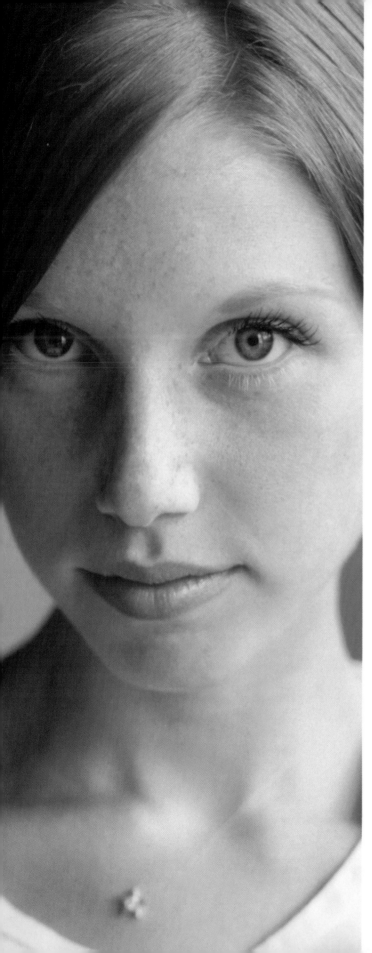

Sincere humility is a beautiful character trait. It's a quality that attracts a lot of attention. You can be good at something and brag about yourself, or you can exercise humility and let others compliment you. If Amanda had been real about her anxieties (which we all experience at one time or another) her teammates would have encouraged her and cheered her on.

In the end, Amanda ended up eating "humble pie" by apologizing to her team for her self-absorbed behavior. The remainder of the season she focused on having a positive attitude, and she encouraged her teammates with praise instead of put-downs. In turn, her teammates gave her the emotional support she needed to be a soccer superstar. In fact, Amanda's humility made such a difference that she was awarded "Most Improved" for her attitude at the school's year-end sports banquet.

The Answer Is

The answer to pride is humility, and humility starts by being real. It might not seem easy at first, but once you let your guard down and start being honest, you'll get a new lease on life. It's like touching your face up with translucent powder; once you apply it, you'll feel refreshed and renewed.

I used to think that people wouldn't like me unless I acted perfect. But what I learned was that they didn't like me until I *stopped* acting perfect. Once I became open and honest, I became approachable. People liked the real me, faults and all!

How did I do it? I tested the waters at first to make sure it would be safe. I started out by stating the obvious. For example, if I made a mistake I took credit instead of trying to blame someone else. From there I advanced to telling the truth without the extreme exaggerations I was prone to make.

I can remember telling a guy that the Nova I was driving was a lender from the garage that was fixing my Ferrari. Can you imagine a sixteen-year-old with her very own Ferrari? Well, I guess anything's possible, but not in my case. Have you ever heard the saying, "If I could buy her for what she's worth and sell her for what she thinks she's worth I'd make a fortune"? The persona I had built around myself was worthless, and the only way I could like myself and have others like me was to tear it down.

We're always at ease around those who know us well, because there's nothing to hide and we can be ourselves. My best friend in high school knew everything about me and liked me for who I was, not who I made myself out to be. She didn't care that I wasn't rich, or that I didn't drive a Ferrari and shop at expensive department stores. I didn't have to impress her; I only had to be honest with her.

Forming perfect friendships doesn't require perfect people. Lasting friendships are based upon enjoying the good times and working through the bad ones together. Being real is what it's all about. This doesn't mean you need to broadcast your faults over the school intercom, but you do need to be honest with your own circle of friends so that you can be accountable to each other. Transparency protects you from superficial relationships.

Lauren was miserable at home. Her parents were getting a divorce, and she was especially embarrassed because her dad was a local public figure. Had she not had friends to lean on during that time, she might have resorted to drugs as a temporary source of relief. But instead she confided in her friends who helped her get through it and kept her accountable for her actions.

Problems, whether big or small, are never too trivial for true friends. Whenever I was in trouble, my friend was the first one I called. I knew I could confide in her without her telling anyone else. Trust is very necessary between friends. If someone tells you something in private, you should never divulge their secret without their permission, unless it could save their life. But don't keep unhealthy secrets about drug, alcohol, or sexual abuse. If you know someone who could hurt herself or someone else, suggest that

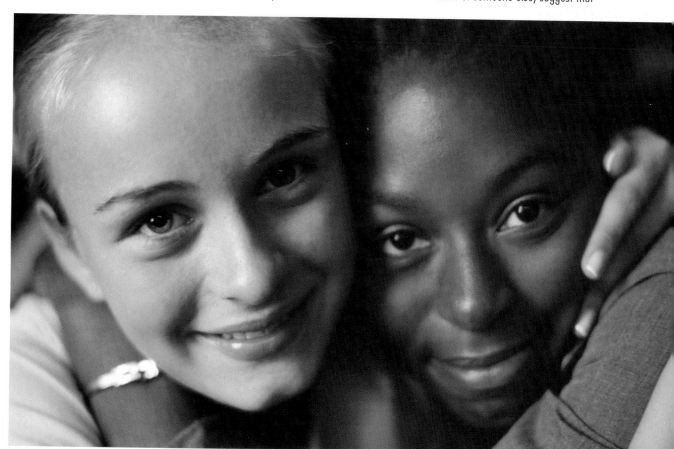

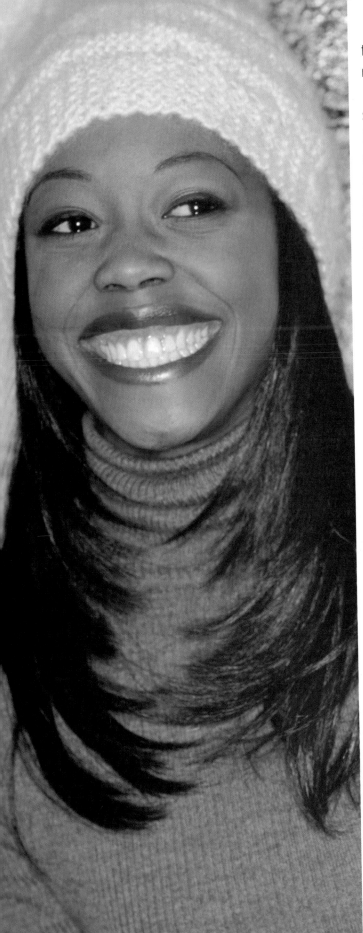

they get help, and if they won't listen, get help for them. They might get mad, but it's better than the alternative.

As a teen, popularity and self-importance can plague your life. It seems like everything revolves around climbing the popularity ladder so that your peers love you. But before you head up, make sure your ladder is set on the right principles so you don't fall down. Secure it in humility, brace it with honesty, and then call on trustworthy friends to hold it in place. And last but not least, don't let pride cause you to look down on others—instead, use your skills to build up someone else.

Beauty Bonus

Not all pride is bad. It's okay to take pride in what you do as long as you do it without being arrogant and boastful.

Amanda learned this lesson the hard way. It took the humiliation of apologizing to her team to understand the importance of having a humble attitude. She then began demonstrating healthy pride in her soccer by practicing and building her skills without being arrogant about her accomplishments. She learned how to inspire others without appearing like an obnoxious know-it-all.

I can't emphasize enough the importance of taking pride in yourself by setting the standard of excellence in all that you do. Do you have a book report to write? Then do it with a certain amount of class and finesse, putting everything you've got into making it your personal best. Do you work at the local burger joint? Then flip those burgers with pride and make your employer happy he hired you, even if you don't like the job. And of course there are always those chores at home that could be done with an attitude of gratitude instead of griping. Make the most of who you are by taking pride in your work and being the best that you can be.

How It Applies

James 4:10—Humble yourselves before the Lord, and he will lift you up.

If we do a reality check, we'll find there is nothing we own bragging rights to. Everything we have, including our talents, is from God. We only possess what he's allowed us to have, and when we humbly acknowledge this, he will respond by bringing honor our way.

Putting It to the Test

Get humble. Get honest. Get real.

It may seem like bragging turns people on to you, but it actually turns them off. Examine who you are from the inside out. If pride is an issue, deal with it before it deals with you. Pretending to be something you're not only gets you in trouble.

Like cheap imitation perfumes, exaggerated claims may attract people to you at first, but after a couple of encounters, they'll realize you don't live up to your claims. You're an original. God didn't make anybody else exactly like you, but that doesn't mean you're not likeable. Give humility and honesty a try. I think you'll discover that you like the *real* you better!

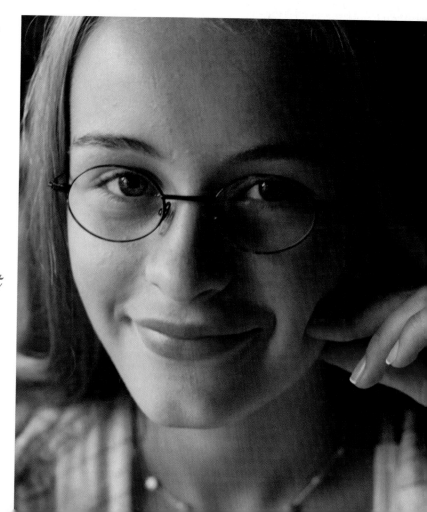

Beauty Secret # 10
Reveal the real translucent
"Super Model" in you.

Tammy's Tip
Take pride in yourself by being all that you can be and doing the best that you can do.

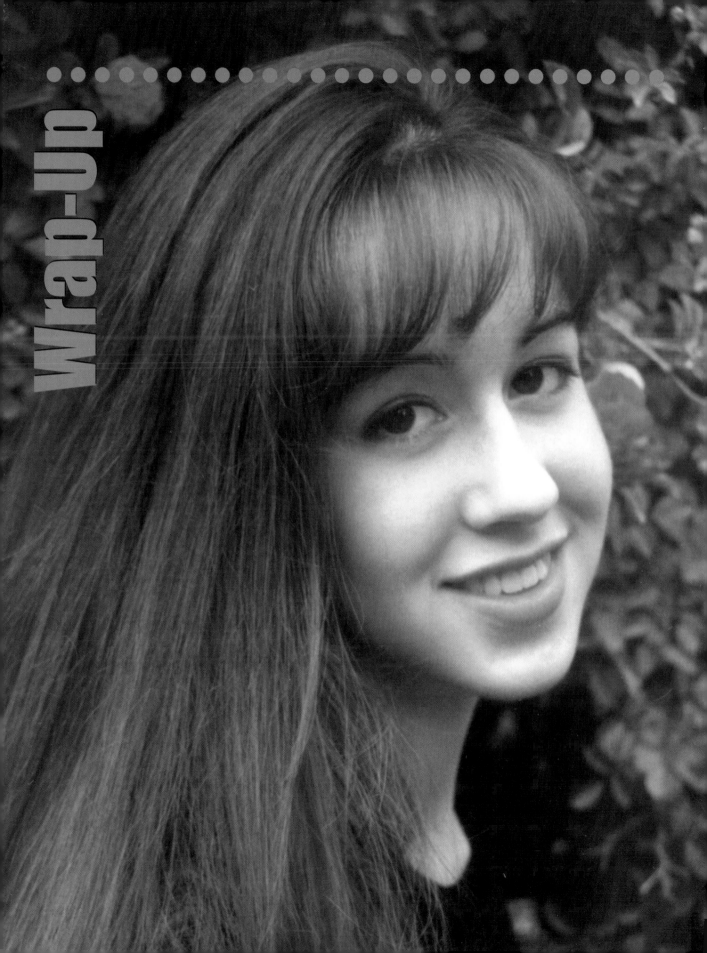

Wrap-Up

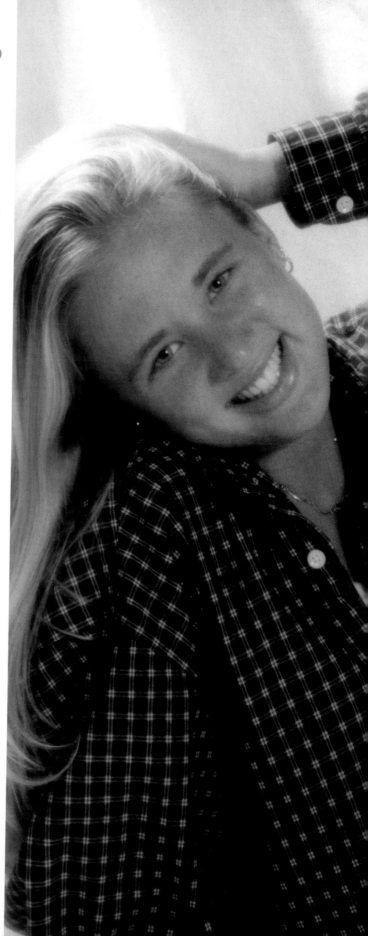

| **'ll try to spare you from a long boring conclusion and wrap it up. I just want to leave you with some quick final words.**

Being beautiful from the inside out is what it's all about. I pray this book has taught you not only how to look great on the outside, but more importantly, how to be beautiful on the inside. True beauty, beauty of the heart and soul, is found on the inside through a relationship with Jesus Christ.

The models you see in magazines have been made over by makeup artists and touched up by graphic artists so that they look perfect on the surface. But what lies beneath all that? Without inner beauty, nothing. You might as well be a photograph, because without a beautiful spirit there is no depth to who you are.

Strive for excellence on the inside first, because being beautiful is not about makeup, hair, or what you wear; it's about who you are on the inside that really counts.

Just as water mirrors your face, so your face mirrors your heart.
Proverbs 27:19 MESSAGE

Be beautiful from the inside out to be a "Super Model."

Final Credits

I couldn't have started, worked on, or finished this book without the love and support of many special people. With deep heart-felt appreciation I want to thank:

My parents for teaching me from an early age about the beauty of my heart through a relationship with Jesus Christ;

My husband Ed, son Matthew, and daughter Ashlee for loving, encouraging, and sticking by me even when I felt like giving up;

Fred and Florence Littauer, who took me under their wings giving me love, nurturing, and guidance through my desert experience and beyond;

My girlfriends, Beth, Rose, Charlotte, Ona, and Jo-Anne for late night gab sessions and much needed advice;

My acquisitions editor, Jennifer Leep, and marketing manager, Twila Bennett, for pouring themselves into this product to make it a complete success;

Josh McDowell, though we met only briefly, your words of encouragement made a lifelong impression;

The CLASS (Christian Leaders, Authors, Speakers Services) staff, for giving me direction in the speaking and publishing world;

The many teens I've had the privilege to counsel and learn life's lessons from;

And finally, my last but certainly most important acknowledgement is to my heavenly Father for inspiring me with a need and a cause to carry out a mission.

I love you all.

Girls, I hope you learn a valuable lesson from these acknowledgements—always say thank you.

Saying Thank You is key to becoming a "Super Model."

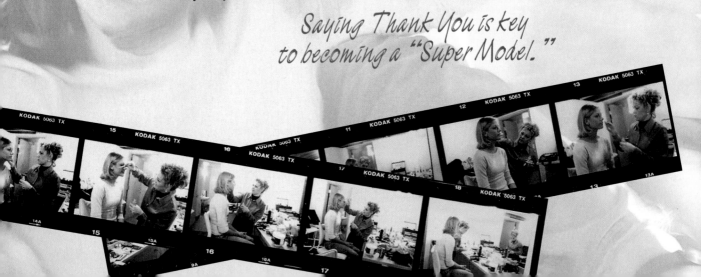